EMDR and Sexual Disorders

EMDR and Sexual Disorders provides fundamental guidelines for the treatment of sexual dysfunctions with EMDR (Eye Movement Desensitization and Reprocessing) within the conceptual framework of attachment theory.

This book demonstrates how the EMDR method, which works specifically on the reprocessing of traumatic memories, can be used to addresses the overall well-being of the patient with the goal of restoring a state of 'sexual health'. The goal is not only the absence of dysfunctions and diseases but also a general condition of physical, emotional, mental and social well-being. After a thorough examination of sexual pathologies and dysfunctions, the authors focus on the traumatic origin of sexual disorders, drawing on extensive clinical experience with victims of abuse and negative attachment stories. A clear and documented picture emerges of how EMDR can provide an innovative and effective contribution to the treatment of pathologies so closely connected to the patient's personal history. The book also introduces two new ground-breaking tools for practitioners: the EMDR protocol for individual sexual dysfunction and the EMDR protocol for sexual dysfunction within couples.

This book offers key essentials to EMDR therapists and any health professional (psychologists, doctors, social workers, etc.) who work in the field of sexology.

Elena Isola, psychologist and psychotherapist, specialises in systemic-relational psychotherapy and clinical sexology. She's an expert in psychotraumatology and in EMDR treatment. She is also a supervisor, child adolescent consultant and facilitator. She's a speaker in national and European congresses on sexological issues and an author of several scientific papers. Her main areas of interest and research concern EMDR therapy, couple's therapy and sexual disorders.

Bruna Maccarrone is a psychologist and psychotherapist specialising in psychotraumatology and EMDR treatment. She is also an EMDR Europe consultant and facilitator, former secretary of the board of the EMDR Italy Association and current chair of the Conference Committee of the EMDR Europe Association.

'This book provides information on sexual disorders for men and women and provides an overview of different treatment methodologies. Then, EMDR therapy is integrated into a wholistic treatment approach. The strength of this book are the case examples that illustrate how the eight phases of EMDR can be applied to various sexual disorders. This book, in a concise way, describes essential information on attachment and dissociation, and a how treatment can be provided within couple therapy, and provides clear case examples. This book is a valuable contribution to the EMDR therapy literature as well as the sexual dysfunction treatment field.'

Roger Solomon, *EMDR Institute, USA*

EMDR and Sexual Disorders

A Practitioner's Guide to Treating Sexual Trauma and Dysfunction

Elena Isola and Bruna Maccarrone

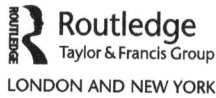
Routledge
Taylor & Francis Group

LONDON AND NEW YORK

Designed cover image: Colorful polygonal people sketches – stock illustration. trendmakers/DigitalVision Vectors via Getty Images.

First published in English 2025
by Routledge
4 Park Square, Milton Park, Abingdon, Oxon OX14 4RN

and by Routledge
605 Third Avenue, New York, NY 10158

Routledge is an imprint of the Taylor & Francis Group, an informa business

Published in Italian as *EMDR e disturbi sessuali* ©2019, Casa Editrice Astrolabio – Ubaldini Editore, Roma.

British Library Cataloguing-in-Publication Data
A catalogue record for this book is available from the British Library

Library of Congress Cataloging-in-Publication Data
Names: Isola, Elena, author. | Maccarrone, Bruna, author.
Title: EMDR and sexual disorders : a practitioner's guide to treating sexual trauma and dysfunction / Elena Isola and Bruna Maccarrone.
Other titles: EMDR e disturbi sessuali. English
Description: Abingdon, Oxon ; New York, NY : Routledge, 2025. | Includes bibliographical references and index.
Identifiers: LCCN 2024036708 (print) | LCCN 2024036709 (ebook) | ISBN 9781032832937 (hardback) | ISBN 9781032825717 (paperback) | ISBN 9781003508670 (ebook) | ISBN 9781040275214 (adobe pdf) | ISBN 9781040275252 (epub)
Subjects: MESH: Eye Movement Desensitization Reprocessing—methods | Sexual Dysfunctions, Psychological—therapy | Sexual Dysfunction, Physiological—therapy | Psychological Trauma—therapy | Sexual Health
Classification: LCC RC556 (print) | LCC RC556 (ebook) | NLM WM 425.5.D4 | DDC 616.85/8306—dc23/eng/20241010
LC record available at https://lccn.loc.gov/2024036708
LC ebook record available at https://lccn.loc.gov/2024036709

ISBN: 978-1-032-83293-7 (hbk)
ISBN: 978-1-032-82571-7 (pbk)
ISBN: 978-1-003-50867-0 (ebk)

DOI: 10.4324/9781003508670

Typeset in Times New Roman
by Apex CoVantage, LLC

Contents

Contributor Biographies

Dr. Paolo Maria Michetti is a highly experienced urologist, sexologist, and researcher, with over three decades of dedication to advancing urological and sexual health. He is a faculty member at the University of Rome "La Sapienza," where he teaches in the fields of urology and surgical andrology across multiple courses and specialties. With over 130 published works and active involvement in international urology societies, Dr. Michetti's research focuses on andrology and oncological urology. He holds specialized certifications in sexology and urology, and his clinical expertise spans from patient care to surgical andrology and rehabilitation.

Dr. Giovanni Simonelli is a distinguished urologist with extensive experience in clinical practice and research. He currently serves as a Medical Director in the Complex Urology Structure at Ospedale Manzoni in Lecco, Italy. Dr. Simonelli has completed his specialization in Urology at Sapienza University, where he also earned his medical degree. He is a member of several professional associations, including the Italian Society of Urology and the European Association of Urology. With numerous publications and conference presentations, Dr. Simonelli is committed to advancing urological care and research.

Foreword

Isabel Fernandez

Sexuality as well as its forms and habits have marked the evolution of the culture of different societies. Different social practices have consolidated in every era with myths, rules and taboos making sexuality one of the most interesting and complex spheres of human life.

From this point of view, the World Health Organisation underlines the centrality of sexuality throughout the life span of the human being, emphasising its many aspects and the possibility of experiencing its various dimensions freely.

Sexology, understood as the study of therapeutic approaches aimed at helping people with sexual issues, could only be a broad and multifaceted subject on the same evolutionary continuum as the object of this study. After the fundamental contribution by the father of psychoanalysis, who, with his work *Three Essays on the Theory of Sexuality*, overcame the common past conceptions of sexuality as a mere adult impulse towards a partner and proposed a theory that contemplates a childhood sexual life, tracing the pathogenesis of sexual dysfunctions in the early years of life, and then, almost a century later, on to cognitive-behavioural therapies and to sex therapy. In this stage, the 'short' approaches to sexual dysfunction mark the birth of intensive treatments to help couples understand how to modify their behaviour and improve the quality of their sexual life. It was not until the 1970s that Helen Kaplan introduced the use of pharmacotherapy in the treatment of sexual dysfunctions, focusing on physiological and personal aspects and not just on the couple's problems. From then on, there was an urgent need to integrate medical, psychological and social aspects into the treatment of sexual problems, customising the cure based on the characteristics of the individual client. The DSM-5 emphasises these aspects well, reminding clinicians of the importance of taking charge of the distress experiences perceived by clients with sexual dysfunctions.

From this point of view, the EMDR, born as an innovative method for the treatment of post-traumatic stress disorders and specialised in the treatment of numerous psychopathologies over the years, could prove to be an effective and targeted intervention in the field of sexology, capable of making an important contribution to the resolution of various dysfunctional aspects of sexuality. Focusing on the different levels (cognitive, emotional and bodily), EMDR becomes a pivotal tool to facilitate the healing of clients, assisting the clinician in the structuring of a therapeutic plan that considers all aspects of suffering, as indicated in the DSM-5.

The objective of this book is to share a good practice in this field of intervention. The authors guide us through the understanding of sexual disorders, explaining the numerous sexual dysfunctions with clear expertise and clinical experience, to be able to understand the mechanisms that underlie these disorders. With a clear and precise writing style, they emphasise the important role of traumatic experiences in the development of sexual disorders, and step by step, they address the different stages of treatment that are indispensable to take care of these clients.

This is an important and innovative book for those who want to work in this field and offers us all the necessary tools to treat sexual dysfunctions in a complete and effective way.

Isabel Fernandez

Isabel Fernandez is a clinical psychologist working in Milan. She is Director of the Psychotraumatology Research Center of Milan and has published many papers, articles and books on trauma, EMDR and other topics. She is the chairman of the Italian EMDR Association and the past president of EMDR Europe Association and a member of the Board of Directors of the Italian Federation of Scientific Psychological Societies.

Foreword

Roger Solomon

EMDR and Sexual Disorders is the EMDR clinician's guide to treating sexual disorders. Since Francine Shapiro's initial discovery of EMDR therapy in 1987, EMDR therapy has come a long way with over 44 randomly controlled studies demonstrating its efficacy for a wide variety of disorders. EMDR therapy is guided by the adaptive information processing model which states that current problems are the result of maladaptively stored memories. EMDR therapy treatment consists of processing the past memories underlying the current problem, presenting triggers and providing a future template for adaptive behaviour. The growth of EMDR therapy is not only in research but also in the clinical application of EMDR to different disorders. The clinician needs to adapt EMDR therapy to each client based on the knowledge and research specific to each disorder. This book provides information on sexual disorders for men and women and provides an overview of different treatment methodologies. Then EMDR therapy is integrated into a wholistic treatment approach. The strength of this book are the case examples that illustrate how the eight phases of EMDR can be applied to various sexual disorders.

Treatment of sexual disorders has to treat not only the sexual problem but also the individual and the couple. The clinician may need to do individual therapy as well as couple therapy. The clinician needs to be knowledgeable about attachment and dissociation, which can underlie sexual difficulties as well as systems theory to provide couple therapy. This book, in a concise way, describes essential information on attachment and dissociation and how treatment can be provided within couple therapy and provides clear case examples.

I have known the senior author, Bruna, for over 20 years. She was one of my first EMDR students when I first came to Italy in 1999 to teach EMDR therapy. I remember well her eagerness to learn, her energy, her enthusiasm, her sense of humour and her excellent clinical abilities. I am so proud of her achievements, having watched her clinical skills, EMDR knowledge and teaching ability grow.

Elena Isola has been active in the field of sexual disorders for over 20 years, conducting research and providing clinical services. After achieving positive clinical results, she started integrating EMDR therapy into treatment of sexual disorders. In conceiving this book, she has enthusiastically and tenaciously pursued her goal to combine and integrate her expertise in clinical sexology and systemic-relational couple therapy with the EMDR therapy approach. Recently, Elena has also become an EMDR supervisor and facilitator.

This book is a valuable contribution to the EMDR therapy literature as well as the sexual dysfunction treatment field.

Roger Solomon, PhD, is a psychologist and psychotherapist specialising in the areas of trauma and grief. He is on the senior faculty of the EMDR Institute and provides basic and advanced EMDR training internationally. He currently consults with the US Senate, NASA and several law enforcement agencies.

Roger Solomon

Introduction

Elena Isola

Over the past few years, the increasingly complex and typical social and cultural changes have highlighted the necessity of an interdisciplinary approach to the treatment of sexual issues, bringing out the need to integrate different medical and scientific disciplines. In other words, the principle according to which 'complex problems' can only be tackled with 'integrated solutions' is deemed as winning in all scientific fields. Of course, even the field of sexology could not avoid this irreversible trend, characterised by important innovations, both with the publication of numerous empirical studies aimed at solving specific clinical aspects and with the introduction of pharmacological proposals effective in treating dysfunctions.

The rapid evolution of sexology as a field is demonstrated by the World Association for Sexual Health's (WAS, 2002) recent update of the definition of 'sexual health' as follows:

> a state of physical, emotional, mental, and social well-being linked to sexuality; not just the absence of disease, dysfunction or infirmity. Sexual health requires a positive and respectful approach to sexuality and sexual relationships, as well as the possibility of having pleasant and safe sexual experiences, free from coercion, discrimination, and violence. In order to achieve and maintain sexual health, the sexual rights of everyone need to be respected, protected and satisfied.

This leads to a more articulated view of sexual behaviour as a psychosomatic unit so that the clinical investigation is required to deal not only with the biological, hormonal, vascular and, in some cases, iatrogenic components of dysfunctions but also with the more strictly psychological and relational aspects of the client, considering the social and cultural context of reference. The purpose of this work is to verify whether it is possible to introduce intervention tools that have proven to be effective in the broader area of psychological care and apply them in the context of sex therapy, concretely leading to an osmosis between different fields of application. Working daily with people who are victims of sexual abuse, or who reported dysfunctional attachment histories, the need has arisen to organise the various aspects of sexual disorders in an overall picture, paying special attention

DOI: 10.4324/9781003508670-1

to the treatment of trauma-based sexual dysfunctions of traumatic origin with the EMDR (Eye Movement Desensitisation and Reprocessing).

This publication is born out of the need to share the direct clinical experience acquired in clinical fieldwork in recent years. The result of research, reflections, questions, attempts and errors.

Born as an innovative technique, EMDR soon became a method and, eventually, a refined and effective psychotherapeutic approach. EMDR uses bilateral alternated stimulation through eye movements or alternating tapping on the back of the hands to unlock and reactivate an innate mechanism of self-healing. This process facilitates the desensitisation and reprocessing of disturbing memories stored in the brain in a partial and dysfunctional manner and that are the cause of various symptoms and/or psychopathological disorders. For this reason, we believe that EMDR can be an effective method of therapeutic intervention in the field of sexology, capable of offering a decisive contribution to the understanding and resolution of various problems of both organic and psychogenic nature.

I would like to thank everyone who supported me personally and professionally in writing this book, firstly, my clients, without whom I would not have been able to learn and fine-tune my intervention strategies.

I would like to thank my father, who helped me in rereading and revising the book with valuable contributions, and Bruna Maccarrone, who believed and supported me during my EMDR training years and for her precious contribution to writing and revising this book.

I would like to thank Isabel Fernandez for her great humanity and professionalism and for the generosity with which she manages the EMDR Association in Italy, offering constant professional and scientific support to the whole community.

Lastly, I would like to thank Paolo Maria Michetti, MD, of the Department of Urology of the University La Sapienza of Rome, who has shown not only great professionalism but also humanity in managing highly traumatised clients with me over the years.

Chapter 1

Sexology and its evolution over time

Elena Isola

1.1 Sexuality

What is sexuality? The definition of the Treccani Encyclopaedia says that it is a 'complex of sexual characteristics and phenomena concerning sex'; hence, it would seem to be a topic that can be categorised clearly. In reality, the subject matter is much more complex, as shown by the official definition of sexuality used by the World Health Organization (WHO):

> Sexuality is a central aspect of the human being throughout life and includes sex, gender identities and roles, sexual orientation, eroticism, pleasure, intimacy and reproduction. Sexuality is hoped for and expressed in thoughts, fantasies, desires, beliefs, attitudes, values, behaviours, practices, roles and relationships. Although sexuality may include all these dimensions, not all of them are always experienced or expressed. Sexuality is influenced by the interplay of biological, psychological, social, economic, political, ethical, legal, historical, religious and spiritual factors.

Therefore, the term 'sexuality' refers to all psychological, social and cultural aspects of human sexual behaviour, while the term 'sexual activity' refers more specifically to the actual sexual practices. The multifaceted and complex character of sexuality emerges in all its strength that is not limited to the fundamental aspect of human behaviour concerning acts aimed at reproduction and the search for pleasure but also ranges over the social aspects connected to it, which have evolved in relation to the different characteristics of the male and female genders.

The history of sexuality is essentially the history of man's awareness towards this essential aspect of life. A long and complex process, far from being completed, which began with the discovery of the reproduction potential for the sexual act that, most likely, occurred in the neo-gothic era. This discovery had a great social importance because it led to the introduction of an increasing number of prohibitions and taboos in the sexual practice, aimed precisely at ensuring the cohesion and survival of the group, through the even drastic regularisation of the sexual drive (Mead, 1991).

DOI: 10.4324/9781003508670-2

Therefore, sexuality is not only an essential characteristic of life but also a qualifying aspect of the evolution of the different human societies adopted over time and that had and have shown considerable differences on this very issue. These considerations are confirmed by the most recent studies reinstating that sexual aspects are of fundamental importance for the construction of personal identity and for the social evolution of the individual:

> Human sexuality is not dictated by instinct or by a behaviour stereotype as with animals, but is influenced, on the one hand, by personal mental activity and on the other by the social, cultural, educational and normative characteristics of those places where individuals develop and create their personality. Therefore, the sexual sphere requires an analysis based on the convergence of various lines of development, including affectivity, emotions, and relationships.
>
> (Boccadoro and Carulli, 2008)

The conclusion we come to is that, in the light of more in-depth knowledge gained over the last few decades, the sexual issue is highly connected to the sphere of human feelings and relationships and includes an emotional and affective background that is of fundamental importance on an individual level and of relevant interest in the social field.

1.2   Sexology and its history

The fact that the study of sexuality is a broad and complex subject is demonstrated by the definition of 'sexology' always provided by the Treccani Encyclopaedia: 'the science of sexuality that includes all the knowledge related to the dynamics between the sexes: gender identity, cultural determinants, couple and family relationships, sexuality, strictly speaking, pathology of relationships and the sexual function'.

The scientific study of sexuality is a relatively recent activity, as it has been greatly conditioned by taboos and social prejudices, in particular, religious ones. The first studies on psychopathological subjects were published at the end of the 19th century by the German psychiatrist R. von Krafft-Ebing (1840–1902) and by the English sexologist H. H. Ellis (1859–1939) and concerned the great variety of sexual perversions, both in the choice of the sexual object and in the type of activity used to obtain satisfaction.

Today, the dermatologist Iwan Bloch is considered the father of modern sexology, seen as an autonomous science, free from conditioning factors such as common sense and religious beliefs. Together with Doctor Magnus Hirschfeld and the neurologist Albert Eulenburg, he founded the first periodical that already included in the header the term he had coined a few years earlier: *Zeitschrift für Sexualwissen schaft* ('*Journal of Sexology*') published in Berlin from 1914 to 1922. According to his effective definition of 'sexology', to assess the global importance of the 'love life' for the individual and for society, as well as for the entire cultural development of mankind, the study of this discipline must integrate with the study of man as such, in collaboration with other disciplines: general biology, anthropology, ethnology, philosophy, psychology, medicine, history of literature and of culture in general (Bloch, 1907).

This conception, in which one cannot but highlight the positiveness of the term 'life of love' for a subject that was object of obtuse prejudice at the time, inspired the development of sexology as a science as we know it today, proposing it as the heritage and object of research of various medical and nonmedical branches and disciplines. Bloch's concept, according to which sexology is a discipline with a marked cultural value and that brings together a wide and vast doctrinal field in which different sciences converge, is extremely valid and topical more than a century after its enunciation.

It is sufficient to mention Rifelli's updated definition, according to which sexology is a non-autonomous discipline that mutates concepts and languages from various other ones. On the other hand, sexuality, which represents its object of study, is equally composite, being a structural set of anatomical, psychological, relational, social and cultural elements. Therefore, a medical, surgical, endocrinological, andrological, gynaecological and psychological sexology exists, but there is also a sociology of sexuality and sexual criminology (Rifelli, 2007).

The history of sexology, in particular, as the study of therapeutic approaches to help people with sexual problems, is rather fascinating. It reflects the global orientations of therapeutic methods used in the treatment of a wide variety of psychological problems for which the emphasis has shifted from the two extremes of pure psychoanalytic treatment and an exclusive physical care to a therapy based on modern psychological principles and on our deeper knowledge of sexuality.

It should be pointed out that in the field of sexology, because of the integrated and interdisciplinary nature of the subject, the following is usually distinguished:

- A biological-medical branch that studies the phenomena of sexuality with respect to genetics and the role of the endocrine and nervous systems in its normal and pathological manifestations;
- A psychological branch, which analyses the dynamics of relational processes, with particular reference to psychoanalytical theories on childhood sexuality and on the maturation of sexuality in the oral, anal and genital phases; and
- A social-anthropological branch that studies the cultural and semiological value of the sexual difference in the social organisation.

Examining the development of modern sexology with a specific reference to the psychological approaches, consistent with the book's topic on the application of the EMDR methodology, three main moments can be identified (Kirana et al., 2013):

- The birth of modern sexology within the European psychoanalytic approach.
- The American development within cognitive-behavioural therapy (CBT).
- Today's international spreading of the biopsychosocial model (BPS).

1.3   The psychoanalytic approach

A fundamental contribution to the development of sexology was made by Sigmund Freud in his work *Three Essays on the Theory of Sexuality* of 1905, in which sexual difficulties are addressed in the psychoanalytic framework, as for the most other psychological symptoms. Freud overcame the common understanding of the term defining sexuality as an instinct – i.e. as a preformed behaviour, characteristic of the species, with a relatively steady partner (usually of the opposite sex) and a target (the union of the genitals in coitus) – because it was inadequate to provide a sufficient explanation, let alone a therapy for sexually related issues. He set up his completely innovative theory affirming that sexology did not only designate the activities and pleasure depending on the functioning of the genital apparatus but also a whole series of excitations and activities, already existing in childhood that give a pleasure irreducible to the satisfaction of a fundamental physiological need (such as those of breathing, nutrition, excretion, etc.) and that are components in the so-called normal form of sexual love. According to Freud, sexual dysfunctions were to be considered symptoms of rooted personality issues originating from early childhood experiences. In fact, he declared that the origin of sexual problems was to be found in maturation disturbances during the different phases of childhood sexuality that interfered with the normal development of the child-parent relationships.

Freud's approach to child sexuality was revolutionary because it not only intended recognising the existence of excitations or early genital needs but also those activities related to the adult's perversions, either because they use somatic zones (erogenous zones) other than the genital zones or because they seek pleasure (e.g. thumb-sucking) independently of exercising a biological function (hence, the concepts of oral and anal sexuality, etc.). Provocatively, Freud preceded his evolutionary theory of sexuality by dealing with perversions extensively. The result was a cross-effect for which anomalies 'normalise' by finding their presuppositions in infantile development, while children's sexuality, characterised by anatomical and functional immaturity, relatively autonomous, sterile and finalised to autoerotic pleasure, was 'perverse and polymorphous'.

The intention of the founder of psychoanalysis was to demonstrate that what appears pathological in the adult is normal for the child. According to Freud, the child is endowed with a precise sexual organisation and sexual energy already at birth. Then a maturation path begins leading to genitality, but it is an experience far from linear. The immature sexual organisations partly evolve spontaneously into the next ones and are partly removed. Childish, partial and anarchic sexual impulses are destined to recede with the barriers of modesty, disgust and morality that society raises for them. If the concept of sexual function or activity has expanded considerably through psychoanalysis, meeting the notion of desire (strictly dependent on a bodily support, the satisfaction of which depends on phantasmatic conditions), seduction and libido, its anthropological connotation, demonstrating the universality of the Oedipus myth (with its correlation, that is the castration complex), has made incest and its prohibition the most general law of marriage and kinship, therefore, the first organising principle of social life.

With these assumptions, the anthropo-analytical approach considers sexuality as present and fundamental in the totality of acts and expressions of human life (childhood and adult, individual and collective, conscious and unconscious, normal and pathological), distinguishing different modalities and factors within sexual determinism: genetic or chromosomal sex, gonadal or hormonal sex, anatomical or body-related sex, social sex, with the function of functional role, phantasmatic or phantasmomic sex, etc. Starting from the concept that sexual symptoms were caused by unresolved conflicts dating back to childhood, in particular, conflicts concerning a problematic attachment or a particular tension towards the parents, the treatment was focused on the 'unveiling' and resolution of the unconscious intrapsychic conflicts underlying the disorder. According to this approach, the symptoms were not addressed directly by the clinician, and psychotherapies were usually very long (Wiederman, 1998; Leiblum, 2007), therefore, expensive and elitist as well as having a mere individual nature. Besides, the literature on the subject showed that the treatment results were unsatisfactory, and a poor attitude towards sexual dysfunction prevailed (Bergler, 1951).

However, sexual difficulties were mainly addressed within the psychoanalytical framework, as for most other psychological symptoms, until the end of the 1960s. Notwithstanding the importance of the psychoanalytic approach in the birth of modern sexology, much criticism has been directed at the Freudian explanatory model in which biological determinism minimised, if not denied, the relevance of social factors. Most confutations have been put forward by female psychoanalysts who, after Freud and in the years of feminism, have tried to elaborate an autonomous developmental pattern of female sexology, with respect to the male pattern that had been the core of Freudian speculation.

Many other issues, such as the onset of sexual drive, its immediate appearance as a perversion of instinct, the loss of the organic purpose, the fact that Freud just postulated a sexology that had virtually existed from the beginning, as well as the debates linking sexual and love choices, have highlighted the need for sexual issues to be the subject of a more and more integrated study, including psychoanalysis, biology, neuroscience, sociology and anthropology.

1.4 Cognitive-behavioural therapy

The overcoming of the psychoanalytic approach began in the late 1950s and early 1960s and led to the affirmation of the cognitive-behavioural therapy – CBT. The first concretisation of the new approach was Warpole's proposal in 1958 of a method based on a systematic awareness as a therapeutic approach to erectile dysfunction and other sexual difficulties. Many reports appeared after this, usually based on the treatment of a few clients consisting in using behavioural therapy methods with quite satisfactory results in the treatment of some sexual problems like 'frigidity' (Lazarus, 1963), vaginism and erectile dysfunction. The introduction of these more directional approaches represented a major conceptual change with respect to the psychoanalytic attitude because treating sexual issues directly concerned current behaviour and its manifestation, rather than distant and hypothetical causes.

A second event was the introduction of a short psychotherapeutic approach in Great Britain based on Michael Balint's teaching for the treatment of sexual problems in women. This approach was of particular interest because it included short psychotherapy strategies and more behavioural-oriented techniques, making it become the hallmark of modern sex therapy. For example, in the treatment of vaginism, a gynaecological examination by the woman's doctor was used for therapeutic purposes to encourage the client to express her anxieties and fears on the vaginal penetration by her partner. These were then explored more deeply to induce and help the woman understand and overcome them. However, it should be noted that an important difference in early behavioural methods compared to modern sex therapy was that the treatment, in these cases, was centred on the individual rather than on the couple; therefore, the partner was excluded from the treatment session. Two studies were particularly relevant in determining the conditions of radical change in sexual therapy, both based on a pragmatic and experimental approach aimed at the physiological aspects of sex. The first was the Kinsey Report, which was the publication of a series of data collected between 1938 and 1952 on the sexual habits of Americans. These publications were much debated at the time because they opened doors to the public and science world of the time that had rarely been explored before then. It was a rather important social study for the time because it displayed sexuality as an important and vital function for human beings, overcoming cultural reluctance and, above all, proposing a 'right to asylum' to female sexuality that was not particularly taken into consideration then.

The second very important event was the publication in 1966 of the book *Human Sexual Response* by the American gynaecologist William H. Masters in collaboration with Virginia Eshelman Johnson, the result of an extensive study on the physiology of sexual intercourse that started in 1954. The social resonance of this book was very great in the Western world and was much debated at the time for two main reasons: whether or not science should enter an intimate area with its sometimes controversial and questionable tools of investigation and the relevance of female sexual activity that was also claimed by the feminist movement in those years. The two scholars followed an innovative approach, largely based on in-depth investigations on the sexual response in men and women, developing a single combination of behavioural, psychotherapeutic and educational elements that provided a relatively direct approach to the treatment of sexual problems in couples.

In contrast to the psychoanalytic approach, Masters and Johnson issued the first proposal on the 'short' treatment for sexual dysfunction, marking the date of birth of sexual therapy: the intensive, time-limited treatment was directed at the symptom and provided for the prescription of behavioural tasks to do separately and a communication training for the couple to reduce performance anxiety and restore a 'natural' sexual response. Masters and Johnson's sex therapy adhered mainly to CBT, with the inclusion of some elements from psychodynamics, educational psychology and communication techniques (Almas and Landmark, 2010).

The theoretical model of the CBT postulated that the behaviours and emotional reactions were learned during development.

The purpose of the therapy was to help people understand how to change their behaviour in order to facilitate an improvement in their feelings and emotions. With the historical example of Masters and Johnson, the requesting couple resided in the clinic for a period of 2–3 weeks, and the therapist proposed some sensory and sexual experiences with the aim of making the couple experience pleasant sexual moments that would change their attitudes and unlock any issues in the various phases of the sexual response (Kirana *et al.*, 2013). The results of the treatment of a large number of couples made known by Masters and Johnson were quite extraordinary, and although subject to much criticism, they gave origin to the enormous enthusiasm that rapidly developed around 'sex therapy' as it is known, both in the United States and elsewhere, even if the implementation of this kind of approach by untrained therapists discredited the system over time. It must be said that the Masters and Johnson method, being intended for couples, effectively excluded single people with sexual problems. Consequently, a more realistic attitude prevails today over the effectiveness of this sexual therapy.

The cognitive-behavioural school reached maturity through the work of Helen Kaplan, who introduced her version of sex therapy born from a combination of different psychotherapeutic approaches (psychodynamic, CBT and systemic relational) and the *ad hoc* use of pharmacotherapy. This way, some of the guiding elements and tasks of the Masters and Johnson's protocol, the more individual and profound aspects of the psychodynamic matrix and the basic concepts of the theory of systems were integrated. In particular, the systemic perspective shifted the focus of sex therapy from the individual to the relationship, concentrating on interpersonal dynamics and interaction models within the couple. From then on, sexual problems were also seen as mainly relational difficulties to be explained within the dynamics of the specific couple (Jurich and Myers-Bowman, 1998; Kirana *et al.*, 2013).

With the Kaplan model, the experience of pleasure and the possibility of re-elaboration of one's own bodily experience gained a space for discussion, without neglecting the medical framework and the use of drugs. For a long time, this model continued to be a cornerstone of clinical sexology and the first form of an international approach to sexual issues.

1.5 The biopsychosocial model (BPS)

In the same years, the need to explain the sexual pathology using a multifactorial perspective was also felt in the medical field. The first to introduce a theoretical model on diseases in the sexual field was Engel (1977), who hypothesised that the genesis of the pathologies should be traced in the interaction of different biological, psychological and social factors.

According to this model, the combination of all these factors leads to the definition of the 'state of well-being' of the person through a concatenation of effects to which the subjective conditions of the client directly contribute.

The BPS model proposed by Engel goes beyond the centuries-old medical view that interpreted the pathology as the result of a simple cause-effect relationship caused by a biological aetiological factor, in which the interaction between health and disease is mechanistic. Vice versa, the proposed system derives from the general theory of complex systems and places the sick individual at the centre of a wide system but influenced by multiple variables. To understand and solve the disease, the physician needs to pay attention to the individual's psychological, social and family aspects, interacting with each other and able to influence the evolution of the disease (Engel, 1977; Becchi and Carulli, 2009).

The concept of 'psychobiological unity' of the human being requires that the physician accept responsibility for assessing any problems the client may have and recommending a series of measures, including referring them to other professionals. Consequently, the physician's basic professional knowledge and skills must include social and psychological aspects as well as biological aspects in order to act in the interest of the client involved in all three of these issues (Engel, 1977). The basic concepts of this model have spread quickly in the health care field, to the point of permeating clinical sexology as well. The BPS model is based on the concept that biological factors (physiology, somatic symptomatology and body manifestations), psychological factors (thoughts, emotions and behaviours) and social factors (economic, environmental, relational and cultural) all have a significant role in human functioning, with regard to both health and disease.

This conception leads to rejecting the unimodal approach that prescribes only biomedical or psychosocial treatment for a sexual problem. Since the origin and outcome of any sexual disorder depends on a combination of these factors, the treatment must necessarily take them into account. The therapist is obliged to observe and analyse the impact of biology, psyche and social environment on the symptom, and their interaction, in the relationship with the client. The challenge the clinician needs to face is empathically finding the significant connections between the client's history and the difficulties he or she brings to the evaluation (Engel, 1997). It should be recalled that the numerous advances made in recent years in the field of sexual medicine have changed the way sexual dysfunction is understood and treated in clinical practice.

The great conceptual revolution is represented by the introduction of phosphodiesterase type 5 (pde-5) inhibitors in 1998 that stimulated a positive attention towards sexual functioning and improved men's and women's perspectives on sexual satisfaction throughout their lives. In addition to pde-5 inhibitors, other drugs have been introduced and used within sex medicine like the selective inhibitors of serotonin reuptake, used in the treatment of premature ejaculation, as well as flibanserin and bremelanotide for female dysfunctions (not available in Italy yet). However, it should be noted that the introduction of these drugs has not eliminated the need for psychosexual therapies that still have a central role as a tool for the successful treatment of sexual dysfunctions (Althof, 2010).

Evidence that medical treatment alone cannot solve all psychological and psychosocial aspects of sexual dysfunction has increasingly opened the door to a BPS model in contemporary sexology. The personal and relational experience of the sexual symptom, as also underlined by the DSM-5 (Diagnostic and Statistical Manual of Mental Disorders) of the American Psychiatric Association, is one of the most important elements that the clinician must evaluate and deal with. Specifically, great importance is given to the perceived distress with respect to the sexual symptoms (Althof, 2010). This approach not only looks at the resolution of the dysfunction but also at the more general concept of the improvement of the quality of life, a central objective for those working in the health care sector according to a BPS vision (Tripodi *et al.*, 2016). Moreover, it is in the facts that the BPS model is functional for the sexual dysfunction therapy and in the very nature of sexuality, which consists in the integration of bodies, feelings, emotions, beliefs, cultures, thoughts, experiences, desires and fantasies, on their own or in relation to one another.

For this, it is not surprising that sexual therapy naturally evolves towards the BPS model that considers the different levels of assessment of the symptoms. It is only reasonable that such an interconnected problem should be tackled with a synergetic approach in therapeutic terms, based on a diversified combination of treatments, adapted and customised to the individual's needs.

The publication of this book stems from the knowledge of this need and from the desire to share positive experiences in the application of EMDR in the treatment of sexual dysfunctions, just as a contribution to the diffusion of psychological practices that can be an integral part of the broader system of intervention, according to the biopsychosocial model approach.

Chapter 2

Sexual disorders

Elena Isola

2.1 General information on sexual disorders

Initially, the authors of the American Psychiatric Association (APA) referred to the distinctions proposed by the sexual pioneers in the DSM, inserting some changes from time to time, reaching the final draft of the DSM-5 that, instead, made significant changes for the clinic.

What does 'sexual dysfunction' stand for? A sexual dysfunction is characterised by an anomaly in the process underlying the sexual response or pain associated with sexual intercourse. These disorders may occur in one or more of the aforementioned stages. The assessment should be made considering age, experience, frequency and chronicity of the symptom, subjective discomfort and influence in other areas of the person's functioning (Fulceri *et al.*, 2016). The *DSM-5* (American Psychiatric Association, 2013) has radically revised, with respect to the previous version (American Psychiatric Association, 1994), the placement and diagnostic definition of the so-called sexual disorders and proposed a comprehension of these disorders in the light of clinical and scientific developments in recent times. In fact, *sexual disorders* are no longer included in the same category in the *DSM-5* but in three distinct categories: *sexual dysfunction, gender dysphoria, paraphilic disorders.*

Regarding the first, a significant change in the classification of sexual dysfunction was the natural consequence of criticism to the assessment of the sexual response in phases (desire, arousal, orgasm). Attention to the sexual response cycle that, in the previous edition of the manual, determined the grouping of dysfunctions into three areas (desire, arousal and orgasm) was strongly weakened (Sungur and Gündüz, 2014). On the contrary, recent literature has shown that the sexual response is not a linear and uniform process and the distinction of the disorders according to phases (e.g. desire and arousal) could be artificial.

In *DSM-5*, there was a need to use more precise definitions, both in terms of time and for the functioning mechanism involved, apt to differentiate a sexual disorder from a transient one (Sungur and Gündüz, 2014). Another important aspect is that up to *DSM-5*, the sexual response was considered similar in the different genders, while scientific literature agrees that sexual interest, motivation, arousal

DOI: 10.4324/9781003508670-3

and pleasure can be experienced more and more differently in the two genders (Sungur and Gündüz, 2014).

Regarding female sexual dysfunctions, sexual desire disorders and sexual arousal disorders merged into one disorder: female sexual interest/arousal disorder. Vaginism and dyspareunia, often coexisting and difficult to distinguish, were incorporated into genito-pelvic pain/penetration disorder. The idea to combine them into a single disorder was dictated by the real difficulty of differentiating these two disorders in clinical practice. The female orgasm disorder is unchanged.

The new classification for men includes hypoactive sexual desire disorder, introduced again for men, delayed ejaculation (formerly known as the male orgasm disorder), erectile disorder that has rightly lost the 'male' adjective and the premature (early) ejaculation that has remained unchanged. Male dyspareunia or sexual pain has disappeared from the manual. The diagnosis of sexual aversion disorder has been eliminated because it is very rarely used and because of the lack of supporting research data. In order to increase diagnostic accuracy and reduce overestimates attached to transient sexual problems, the dysfunctions must last at least six months, except the ones that are secondary to substance use. These changes provide thresholds for making a diagnosis and distinguish transient sexual difficulties from more persistent dysfunctions. However, once again, the recommendation is to consider sexual symptoms as mental disorders only after excluding any organic component. Therefore, collaboration between specialists enhanced further (Signorelli, 2014).

Only two subtypes are used to identify the start of the difficulty: permanent/acquired and generalised/situational:

• 'Permanent' if there is a sexual problem from the first sexual experiences;
• 'Acquired' if sexual disorders develop after a period of normal sexual performance;
• 'Generalised' if the sexual difficulties are not limited to specific types of stimulation, situations or partners; and
• 'Situational' if the sexual difficulties occur only with certain types of stimulation, situation or partner.

The *DSM*-5 also takes a number of factors into account (indicated as associated characteristics) that may be relevant both for the aetiology and for the treatment of the sexual disorder, such as the following: 1) factors concerning the partner, 2) relationship difficulties, 3) individual psychological vulnerability factors (e.g. stories of sexual or emotional abuse or unsatisfactory body image) as well as comorbidity with other symptoms (depression, anxiety) or stressful factors (job loss, mourning), 4) cultural and religious factors and, finally, 5) relevant medical factors.

Significant changes for the adequate classification of these disorders, which further confirm their multidimensional matrix, implicitly recognised with the same definition reported in the manual, are as follows: 'The sexual response is fundamentally biological but is generally experienced in an intrapersonal, interpersonal and cultural context: therefore, the sexual function implies a complex interaction between biological, socio-cultural and psychological factors' (American Psychiatric Association, 2013, page 494). A scale measuring the severity of the disorder – mild, moderate or severe – has also been included. The term 'due to psychological factors or a combination of factors' was suppressed since the APA judged this differentiation as a false dichotomy between psychological and oral disorders, both of which are often present.

A new exclusion criterion was introduced: the disorder should not be explained as a 'psychic disorder that does not have a sexual nature' nor as a consequence of a particularly stressful couple relationship, and there should be no other particularly stressful conditions. Therefore, if the sexual dysfunction depends on a psychic disorder other than a typical sexual problem, the diagnosis cannot be made. Finally, this new edition of *DSM-5*, beyond the limits and controversies inherent to the conceptual aspects, underlines the importance of the distress criterion, the subjective discomfort that the client feels. This concept, existing since the DSM-III, was added to the current edition in 46% of all Axis I and II disorders and specifically in all sexual dysfunctions (Hendrickx *et al.*, 2013). The importance given to the evaluation of distress in the diagnosis of sexual dysfunction shows the importance of the subjective and relational aspects in this field. Although, in most cases, sexual activity involves at least two partners, many clinicians stress that sexual distress should be considered a disorder when it causes personal distress and when it causes interpersonal difficulties too (Sungur and Gündüz, 2014).

Gender dysphoria is a new diagnostic class of *DSM-5* as a result of a change in the conceptualisation of the characteristics defining the disorder, determined by the suffering that may accompany the inconsistency between the gender experienced or expressed by an individual and the assigned gender. The 'gender incongruence' phenomenon is emphasised instead by the identification with the opposite sex, as had been the gender identity disorder in the previous diagnostic version. The pathology connotation is reduced basically, but mainly, it is the discomfort that accompanies this condition that is recognised. The term 'gender' is systematically used instead of 'sex' because the concept of sex is deemed inadequate when referring to individuals with a sexual development disorder. The current term is more descriptive than the previous term, 'gender identity disorder', because it focuses on dysphoria as a clinical problem and not on the actual identity.

For *paraphilic disorders*, a general change from the previous manual is the addition of 'controlled environment' and 'in remission' course specifiers to the diagnostic criteria for all paraphilic disorders. Their usefulness concerns prognostic and forensic psychiatric implications in particular. In *DSM-5*, paraphilia is not always framed as a minor disorder. It is necessary that this leads to discomfort or impairment of the individual or personal harm or risk of harm to others. 'Paraphilia is a necessary but not sufficient condition for a paraphilic disorder, and paraphilia does not automatically justify, or require, a clinical intervention' (American Psychiatric Association, 2013, p. 947). The paraphilic disorders included in the manual are voyeuristic disorder, exhibitionist disorder, frotteuristic disorder, sexual masochism disorder, sexual sadism disorder, paedophilic disorder, fetishist disorder and transvestism disorder. However, this list does not exhaust all possible paraphilic disorders. Many more different paraphilia forms have been identified, but in order to speak of a real disorder, the negative consequences for the individual and the others must be evaluated (Mantione and Presti, 2016).

2.2   Female sexual disorders

'Sexual dysfunction' is an expression that encloses multiple alterations of the pathophysiology of sexual response, with particular attention to their genital expression. Female sexual dysfunction (FSD, female sexual disorders) can appear in a continuum ranging from dissatisfaction (with potential integrity of the physiological response but emotional-affective frustration), to dysfunction (with or without pathological modification), to the pathology rooted in biology. The FSDs can cause a variable degree of personal and interpersonal distress and suffering. Sociocultural factors can also widely modulate the problem's perception and verbal expression mode. The meaning of sexual intimacy and the problem itself for the woman and the couple greatly influences the experience resulting from it, the prognosis, the adhesion to therapy and the variability of the therapeutic outcome.

Female sexuality is multifactorial and composed of biological, psychosexual and social factors linked to the woman's social and couple context and is therefore discontinuous throughout her life (Dennerstein et al., 2006; Basson, 2004; Binik et al., 2002; Aslan, 2008). The incidence of FSD increases with the client's age and is estimated to be between 20% and 43% in fertile age (Graziottin, 2007) and 48% in the post-menopausal period (Dennerstein, 2006). In the last decade, many steps have been taken in the understanding of the neuroanatomical and neurochemical bases of arousal and orgasm, searching, at the same time, for new treatments combining pharmacological and psychotherapy contributions. The interest of clinicians and researchers has focused on the physiology of female sexual response, trying to clarify especially the physiology of pleasure and orgasm. An important contribution is made by the interest of uro-gynaecology in sexuality.

While the interest of gynaecology in this delicate field has increased on the one hand, some psychotherapists have distanced themselves from the prevalent medicalisation of sexual dysfunctions, underlining the specific cultural-historical aspect of female gender identity and the different relational value given to sexuality. Moreover, they have warned against the easy use of drugs of which the relapses are not always known (Simonelli et al., 2003). Many international consensus conferences have been organised in recent years to promote a broad confrontation between various experts and, above all, to favour the study of the nosography and the classification system of sexual problems. These meetings have facilitated communication between different disciplines even if an agreement has not always been reached. The debate concerns whether to consider sexual problems as dysfunctions like with somatic and psychiatric diseases, including them in the diagnostic manuals, or to consider them differently. It is precisely in this direction that Tiefer criticises the tendency towards a diagnostic practice because she states that the inclusion of sexual problems in the Diagnostic and Statistical Manual of Mental Disorders of the APA pathologises the possible normal variations of sexual response and contributes to the formation of a standardised conception of sexuality. The controversy is not easy to solve because if, on the one hand, there is a high risk of a stereotyped and medicalised model of sexuality, on the other hand, a more systematic knowledge of sexual problems allows a more targeted intervention, especially for the clinician.

The first Consensus Development Conference on Female Sexual Dysfunction was held in Boston in 1998 and promoted by the Sexual Function Health Council of the American Foundation for Urologic Disease. One of the objectives of this multidisciplinary meeting was to evaluate and review existing classifications on female sex dysfunctions. The conference led to the proposal for a new classification of female sexual dysfunctions (Basson *et al.*, 2000). Moreover, an essential element of the new diagnostic system is the personal distress criterion included in all pathological categories. In fact, a diagnosis of female sexual dysfunction can be made only if the personal experience related to the disorder is one of suffering; therefore, the indication of the partner or the possible deviance from normative cultural models is not deemed as sufficient (Simonelli *et al.*, 2003).

2.2.1   Classification of female sexual dysfunctions

Most female sexual disorders are related to a specific stage of the sexual response cycle or at least one of them. Female sexual disorders can be of various nature.

Therefore, it is necessary to exclude that sexual disorders can be attributed, completely or in part, to medical causes or to taking medication. The sexual response cycle is established consequently to subjectively effective psychophysical and psychological stimuli; therefore, the anatomical-functional integrity of organs and apparatuses designed to trigger and evolve the sexual reaction is a prerequisite for the sexual function.

Female sexual dysfunctions are be divided into four categories: female sexual desire and arousal disorders, orgasm disorder and disorders related to sexual pain.

2.2.2   Female sexual desire and arousal disorders

The *DSM*-5 establishes that the criteria for diagnosing a *female sexual desire and arousal disorder* are as follows: absent or reduced sexual interest, absence of erotic thoughts or fantasies (as with the old hypoactive sexual desire disorder) and either absent or reduced activity in four aspects of sexual life (beginning of sexual activity or response to the partner's attempt to initiate it, absence of sexual arousal and sexual pleasure, absence of a response to sexual stimuli, absence of sensations, genital or non-genital, during sexual activity). At least three of these criteria are required for a diagnosis of female sexual desire and sexual arousal disorder.

Sexual desire is the most elusive dimension of human sexuality because it is difficult to provide an exact objective definition of it, and above all, it is impossible to obtain a quantitative measure. According to Levine (2003), desire is a central topic in the debates pertaining to natural sciences and the humanities. Much has been theorised about the nature and characteristics of sexual desire from anthropology to physiology. Physiology emphasises the necessary integrity for the neuroendocrine system and its connections to achieve an adequate sexual response. Therefore, desire cannot be traced back to a mere biological function. Much richer and more complex, it is affected by personal history and shows variations and fragility.

Today, there is agreement on the definition of sexual desire as a construct complex to be inserted in a multidimensional perspective. In particular, female desire would be more shaded and less genital than male desire, articulated mainly around the quality of the relationship. Kaplan, in her contribution *sexual desire disorders*, proposed a three-phased model of the sexual response (desire, arousal and orgasm) for the first time, indicating that the desire appetite is the necessary premise for the two subsequent phases already widely identified by the scientific community. However, it was thanks to the contribution of Lief (1997) that the desire disorder was addressed according to a scientific perspective, outlining the possibility of a coherent definition aimed at identifying the diagnostic criteria useful to identify the dysfunctions related to it. Leiblum (2002) argues that how we experience and express our sexual interest is determined by biological and, above all, sociocultural drives, highlighting how women are more influenced by them. The author also points out that women have less interest and more sexual problems than men do. According to Levine (2003), women reach sexual desire after establishing a certain psychological intimacy with a new partner, while men start, much more simply, from the sexual behaviour and then reach an intimacy. The different ways of understanding the needs of sexuality create a space for compromise for couples.

In the last 20 years, the incidence of requests for help for sexual desire disorders has increased significantly (Basson, 2003). Women that were unable to reach pleasure during sexual intercourse were branded as frigid. The concept of frigidity or sexual anaesthesia has long been a term applied to a wide range of inhibitions within a woman's sexual response, ranging from a total lack of response to sexual stimulation to various inadequate orgasmic responses, regardless the fact that sexuality is pleasurable for the woman or not. Kaplan (1979) attributed the lack of arousal to a low sexual desire that, in some forms, can have an organic genesis.

Today, we know that female sexual arousal tends to be more widespread, not limited to the genital area, and more difficult to measure than male arousal. In addition, women have sexual fantasies that involve a greater presence of themes related to affection and commitment. This would lead to a differentiation with respect to stimuli that can trigger sexual arousal reactions. It is interesting to note that women do not tend to consider physical manifestations as a measure of their arousal. Women with a healthy sexual desire suffering from a lack of oestrogen report some dryness and pain or discomfort due to penetration, while they do not complain about any loss of sexual arousal. Vaginal lubrication, considered as the physical signal of female arousal, is not perceived by women as such. Indeed, some believe that excessive stimulation is not attractive and causes discomfort. Female sexual arousal disturbances can occur in at two different levels: a lack of physical change that indicate a state of arousal (vaginal lubrication and vasocongestion, i.e. increased blood flow at the genital level) and a deficiency in the subjective component of sexual pleasure and arousal (lack of the psychological sensation of pleasure).

The most recent studies have made it possible to link this disorder to diabetes, hypertension and smoking, which, in the past, were deemed responsible only for the male dysfunction. Menopause and some hormonal disorders can also be responsible for a dysfunction of female sexual desire and arousal. Many authors agree on the existence of various causes for the inhibition of desire: biological factors like hormonal disorders, depression, drug use and organic diseases; psychosocial factors like various forms of depression, anxiety, stress, the presence of other sexual disorders, sexual trauma, sense of guilt and religious restrictions (Berman *et al.*, 2001; Leiblum *et al.*, 2000; Schnarch, 2000). Loss of desire is frequent in subjects using antihypertensive or antidepressant drugs (Burchardt *et al.*, 2002; Rosen *et al.*, 1999).

The psychological aspects of female sexuality are particularly evident at this stage. The relationship with the partner, the different erotic pleasure modalities, the fear of an unwanted pregnancy, low body awareness and anxiety characterise and modulate the woman's ability to let herself go and appreciate the pleasant sensations that lead to excitement. With regards to the diagnosis and treatment of this female difficulty, there is a tendency to propose an integrated approach that includes both medical interventions and sexual therapy because this dysfunction could be a complex overlapping of physical and psychological causes that need to be considered simultaneously (Harrar & Vantine, 1999). Psychosexual evaluation goes beyond the traditional psychological evaluation and is used to learn about the sexual history of the female client and couple, the current sexual practices, the history and quality of sexual intercourse, emotional health and contextual factors that influence their lives (Althof and Leiblum, 2004).

The first questions in our clinical practice, after the anamnesis pertaining to the social-personal data, are aimed at investigating, first of all, the specific nature of the sexual problem: whether it has always been part of the client's life, if it appeared at a specific time or perhaps in relation to an event or if it occurs always or only with certain partners or in certain situations. The sexual desire and arousal disorder may be *primary* or *secondary*. The first seems to be rather rare and is characterised by a total or almost total absence of sexual desire throughout a person's life, including adolescence, even with a lack of sexual fantasies. The secondary disorder, on the other hand, occurs at a certain point in a person's life after a normal, or at least sufficiently adequate, emotional and sexual development. The sexual desire and sexual disorder arousal can also be divided into global and situational. In the latter case, the disorder is related to specific situations like a particular context or in the relationship with a specific partner. The global disorder, on the other hand, tends to disregard specific contexts and relationships and is a lifelong condition of the person.

The prognosis is less optimistic when the lack of desire and arousal is epiphenomenous of a transitional crisis of the couple and of a loss and/or absence of emotional intimacy. In this case, both partners must agree to question themselves and enter a therapy aimed at a substantial improvement of emotional and erotic intimacy.

2.2.3   Female orgasm disorder

It is defined as a persistent or recurrent difficulty in reaching orgasm, despite adequate stimulation and arousal that causes *personal distress*. The partial or total absence of orgasm is one of the most frequent sexual disorders in women. It is characterised by a selective inhibition of the orgasmic reflex, generalised or limited to certain triggers, i.e. certain types of stimulation/sensation. For example, there may be a clitoral stimulated orgasm but not a coital stimulated one. Orgasm inhibition can be isolated, and therefore, desire, excitement and subsequent pelvic congestion may normally be intact, or anorgasmia may be associated with comorbidity, and therefore a decrease of desire, excitement and/or the presence of sexual pain. Women show a wide variability in the type and intensity of orgasm-inducing stimulation. The female orgasm disorder diagnosis should be based on the clinician's assessment that the woman's ability to orgasm is below the expectation due to age, sexual experience and an adequacy of sexual stimulation received. Female orgasm disorder should occur 75%–100% of the time and should be characterised by an absence or delay in reaching it as well as by its stable rarity. The anomaly causes considerable discomfort or interpersonal difficulties.

Worth mentioning, even if not yet well encoded from the nosographic point of view, is the excessive orgasm disorder, which is mainly a spontaneous orgasm (without sexual stimulation) and/or inappropriate to the context that may not necessarily be sexual.

Orgasmic difficulty is generally reported in 15%–20% of sexually active women. When the analysis distinguishes between different types of orgasm, about 10% of women complain about the absolute inability to have one, while about 50% complain about an inability limited to coital orgasm. The value of female orgasm and the classification of orgasm disorders are a product of history and culture (Heiman, 2000). Various meanings and levels of importance have been attributed to the female orgasm throughout the centuries. The problems found in the study of this sexual response phase are of two types: for those who study its neurophysiological aspects, the difficulty of a direct measurement to document when orgasm occurs and, for all, the absence of a general agreement on a shared subjective definition of orgasm. In fact, some clients report the experience in a confused way because not all women know how to recognise the orgasmic experience. In fact, there can be different types of difficulties ranging from a complete lack of orgasm to a situation of uncertainty or the absence of it during coitus, with the possibility, however, of achieving maximum pleasure outside penetration. It must be taken into account that orgasm problems do not always cause sexual distress or marital unhappiness.

In fact, many women manage to have satisfactory sexual intercourse even without reaching orgasm (Meston and Heiman, 1998).

Besides, the distinction between vaginal and clitoral orgasm is no longer necessary. Physiology studies comfort women that have always experienced difficulties in reaching orgasm through coital intercourse, as both experiences are mainly induced by clitoral stimulation (Hirsch, 1998; Masters and Johnson, 1970).

According to the multidisciplinary working group, formed by international experts, promoted by the *Sexual Function Health Council of the American Foundation for Urologic Disease*, orgasm disorder can be defined as the delay or absence of orgasm attainment, despite stimulation and excitement, and must be a source of personal distress (Basson *et al.*, 2000). Later on, Basson *et al.* (2003, 2004) delved into the concept by considering the orgasm disorder in woman as 'lack of orgasm, markedly reduced intensity of orgasmic sensations or marked delay of orgasm in response to any kind of sexual arousal, despite a high level of subjective sexual arousal'. The latter aspect, which was absent in *DSM IV-TR* (2000), subverts the idea that had been widely accepted by experts and that considered the orgasm disorder as due to inadequate sexual arousal; orgasm disorder deserves a diagnostic placement only when it exists despite adequate physical and psychic arousal (Leiblum and Graziottin, 2004). According to some epidemiological studies, orgasm problems are in second place for female sexual dysfunction (Laumann *et al.*, 1999).

As with other sexual dysfunctions, an accurate distinction between primary and secondary anorgasmia is essential at the time of diagnosis for the planning and prognosis. Women who suffer from difficulties in reaching orgasm should be treated in a multidisciplinary way taking into account organic, psychological and relational aspects at the same time. Caution should be exercised when defining orgasmic problems as physical or psychic because there is actually a continuous interaction between various factors: experience, history, previous relationships and culture continuously interact with neurophysiology (Heiman, 1998). Among the neurophysiological factors responsible for the dysfunction, vascular insufficiency seems to have a leading role, but there is still little data supporting this hypothesis (Goldstein and Berman, 1998).

According to Laumann and collaborators, significant factors seem to be education, marital status and age. Among the psychosocial factors, anxiety in various forms has a fundamental inhibitory role, contributing to the loss of concentration on one's sexual sensations. There are no consistent results to support a set of factors that can discriminate between orgasmic and non-orgasmic women. Wiederman (1997) conducted a study on women faking orgasm during coitus. Fifty-five percent of those surveyed claimed to fake orgasm as a habit during sexual intercourse. The author argues that this tendency can be explained by the need to be considered as good sexual partners. However, clinical experience suggests that women also maintain a strong expectation of having to reach orgasm with penetration, perhaps because this relationship mode is considered as the most important (Simonelli *et al.*, 1998). Hite (1998) deems that women are able to experience their sexuality more freely only when they are aware that reaching orgasm through clitoral stimulation does not necessarily mean that they are just content or have sexual problems.

Actually, there can be different kinds of requests for help ranging from a complete lack of orgasm to a situation of uncertainty or absence of coitus, with the possibility, however, of achieving maximum pleasure without penetration.

The aetiology of orgasm disorders can be multifactorial and multisystemic (Franzese, 2015); therefore, the following factors should be considered:

Biological factors

(a) Hormonal: as a result of the absolute or relative deficiency of androgens, and therefore with a block to the genital orgasmic response, in particular, clitoral and vestibular bulb, for the reduction of the responsiveness of the corpus cavernosum smooth muscle.

- Oestrogens, for the inadequate preparation of the orgasmic platform, especially in the form of the congested perivaginal and periurethral vascular tissues.

(b) Ageing-dependent: the histologically documented reduction of about 50% of the smooth muscle component of the corpus cavernosum from the first to the sixth decade of life may be a poorly diagnosed factor in impoverishing the quality of the orgasm both in terms of the time and intensity of stimulation needed to reach it and in terms of the intensity of the sensations and the number of muscle contractions associated with the actual orgasm.

(c) Dystrophic: especially when the *lichen sclerosus* forms involve all the thickness, including the vestibular and clitoral bulb-cavernous structures.

(d) Iatrogens: due to the side effect of the following:

- Drugs, in particular, for the effect of the famous antidepressants and of the type of selective serotonin reuptake inhibitors (SSRI) and tricyclics; sometimes even antiandrogens can cause the orgasm selective (and reversible) inhibition;
- Surgery that has injured the pudendal nerve (reducing sensory afference) or hyperzelant colpoplasty that, by causing a reduction of the vaginal habitability and, therefore, dyspareunia, can also reflexively inhibit arousal, the formation of the orgasmic platform and, therefore, also reaching orgasm;
- Obstetric surgery (surgical births with forceps and/or suction cups), births with macrosome fetuses, or posterior rotation of the occiput, and/or prolonged expulsive periods, i.e. all conditions in which the medial parts of the levator ani muscle have been injured and that are in charge with the efferent, muscular and, therefore, motor complement of the orgasmic reflex. Childbirth and obstetric damage are the most frequent cause of acquired coital anorgasmia, secondary to hypotonia, of varying severity, of the levator ani. The frequent episodes with incomplete reconstruction should also

be mentioned. Clinically, this can cause a diagnostic disorder of vaginal hypoesthesia; and

- Pelvic radiotherapy, for cervical, or anal, or bladder carcinomas that can inhibit orgasm in a complex mode (from vasculopathy and neuropathy) to which the inhibitory effect reflected by dyspareunia for the reduced lubrication and reduced vaginal habitability must be added.

(e) Toxicological: alcohol or drugs, like marijuana, morphine or heroin that, with varying degrees of potency, depress the activity of the central nervous system and can inhibit orgasm through a sedative action on both desire and mental arousal, especially in chronic abuse. Initially, alcohol and marijuana, due to their mild anxiolytic effect, can ease orgasm (because they can reduce the performance anxiety through a general uninhibition effect).

(f) Neurological: e.g. from multiple sclerosis that can impair the nervous component of the orgasm.

(g) Muscular:

- From marked hypotonia, rarely primary, usually secondary, especially obstetric trauma; and
- Hypertonia due to a reflex inhibition caused by pain during the penetration attempts.

(h) Traumatic:

- Accidental: for falls not only with clitoral trauma but also with coccygeal trauma. In this case, it is possible to have a compressive pudendal syndrome (S2-S3-S4) that can occur even years after the trauma, with a deficit of orgasm, as well as vulvar paraesthesia and clitoralgia;
- Sportspeople, with chronic micro-traumas: a chronic compressive pudendal syndrome, described for female cyclists (but also spinning lovers) as well as male cyclists, can cause an impoverishment of the orgasmic quality, as well as genital paraesthesia; and
- Rituals: infibulation, with varying degrees of injury to the clitoris and bulbovestibular structures, can cause a partial or total injury to the genital orgasmic capacity, especially for clitoral stimulation.

(i) Vascular and dysmetabolic:

- Smoking, arteriosclerosis and hypertension can cause a comorbidity between arousal and orgasm disorders, as, in severe forms of damage, they may not allow the formation of an adequate orgasmic platform.
- Diabetes can cause orgasmic damage to the neuropathy characterising it and can complicate the damage on arousal and orgasm secondary to microangiopathy, especially in conditions of a chronic bad glycaemic control.
- Clitoral priapism, generally due to idiopathic cause, can cause anorgasmia, as genital sexual stimulation is intolerable because of the clitoralgia characterising it.

(l) Urological: from detrusorial instability or an overactive bladder that causes an urgency incontinence to orgasm: many clients refer a selective inhibition of orgasm due to the fear that urine loss continues.

Psychosexual factors

*   Erotic illiteracy and sexual inhibition are the main causes of primary anorgasmia.
*   Depression, chronic stress and performance anxiety are the main functional causes of secondary anorgasmia.

Context-related factors

Conflict in a couple, unsatisfactory intimacy and verbal or physical abuse can cause selective inhibition of orgasm or a more aggressive disinvestment from sexual intimacy.

Lack of orgasm can be either primary (if orgasm has never been perceived in any form, including sleep-dreaming orgasms, voluntary and involuntary sexual fantasies, autoeroticism and various types of sexual intercourse) or secondary (if occurring after a period of normal responsiveness and is, therefore, acquired). It can also be either absolute (no form of orgasm ever perceived, in no situation and with no partner; therefore, it is a generalised impossibility) or relative (limited to one aspect of stimulation, one situation and/or one partner). This disorder is referred most frequently during consultations. In fact, many women have nocturnal orgasms during sleep with dreams but are unable to have them with clitoral stimulation and/or penetration. Others have an easy clitoral response but not vaginal or anal.

The adequacy of the diagnostic, anamnestic and semeiological approach to orgasmic disorder will guide the choice of any instrumental examination and the therapeutic, medical, rehabilitative, psychosexual or relational strategy. Orgasm disorders, like all sexual disorders, acknowledge complex causes: biological, psychosexual and relational. Psychosexual and relational factors are related to young women more frequently, including the erotic illiteracy of partners. In orgasm disorders, the likelihood of an increasingly rooted disorder on the biological front increases with age, particularly in acquired forms. This requires new attention on the medical sexuality front due to the growing comorbidity between urological, gynaecological, proctologic and psychiatric diseases and sexual disorders in women.

2.2.4 Genito-pelvic pain and penetration disorder

Part of this dysfunctional area are those disorders that cause a feeling of pain during intercourse. According to traditional classifications, there was talk of dyspareunia and vaginism, but the recent contribution of Basson (2000) invites to extend this dysfunctional area to non-coital sexual pain disorders.

The *DSM*-5 reports that the fundamental manifestation of *genito-pelvic pain disorder and penetration* consists of one or more of the following problems:

difficulty in vaginal penetration during intercourse; marked vulvo-vaginal or pelvic pain during intercourse or attempts at vaginal penetration; marked fear or anxiety about pelvic or vulvo-vaginal pain before, during or as a result of vaginal penetration or marked tension or contraction of pelvic floor muscles during vaginal penetration attempts. In DSM-5, there is a merging of the diagnoses of dyspareunia and vaginism into a single entry called genital-pelvic pain and penetration disorder. This decision was based on the fact that the two disorders cannot be reliably differentiated for two main reasons. First, the formulation of the diagnosis of vaginism as 'vaginal muscle spasm' was not supported by sufficient empirical evidence. Secondly, fear of pain or fear of penetration are common in clinical descriptions of vaginism. Kaplan speaks of it as a 'phobic avoidance', but Carvalho *et al.* (2014) believes that the diagnoses of vaginism and dyspareunia are very often overlapping.

There are clinical studies suggesting a high degree of comorbidity for vaginism and dyspareunia, and many gynaecological studies question the validity of the distinction (Basson and Riley, 1994; van Lankved *et al.*, 1995). A consequence of merging the two diagnoses is the deletion of male dyspareunia, especially since it is considered extremely rare.

The ethology of genito-pelvic pain disorder and penetration in most cases is as follows:

a) Multifactorial, as biological, psychosexual and relational factors (or context-dependent, in the broadest sense) can contribute to this symptom.
b) Multisystemic, in the sense that the complex sexual function requires the integrity of multiple systems: nervous, especially in the central and peripheral pain system, endocrine, vascular, immune and muscular systems; and the integrity of colon and vaginal ecosystems. Pain itself involves multiple biological systems.
c) Complex, in the sense that the resulting functional and overall experience is more than the sum of the individual biological, psychological, sexual and relational parts (Franzese, 2015).

In clinical reality, biological and psychosexual aspects are usually weaved. What varies is the relative proportion, the specific weight of each variable in the clinical picture that each woman takes to the consultation. Psychosexual and relational factors always translate into neurobiological alterations due to the interdependence between psychoplasticity and neuroplasticity. There is no psychic expression without millions of neurons interacting with each other. For example, fear of pain can inhibit sexual availability, through the braking that the anxiety-fear system exerts on the appetite circuits of desire and the parallel over-activation of the adrenergic system that inhibits genital arousal through vasoconstriction. Seat and characteristics of pain, and characteristics of its onset, are the most important predictive factors of the organic aetiology of the genito-pelvic disorder.

An accurate anamnesis and careful physical examination to diagnose and accurately describe the 'pain map' are essential for the diagnosis, and the following need to be investigated:

1) The seat of pain, carefully examining possible points of pain:

- Introital: from vestibulitis, vaginism, neurogenic hyperalgesia of the pudendal, retracting episiotomy scars, iatrogenic outcomes of vaginal surgery (hyperzelant colpoplasty), vulvodinitis;
- Vaginal-lateral medial: from levator hypertonia to myalgia with tender and/or trigger points.
- Vaginal-anterior medial: from cystalgia, trigonite and urethritis.
- Introital and posterior mediovaginal: from fissures, iatrogenic haemorrhoidectomy outcomes, anism; and
- Deep vaginal: from endometriosis, pelvic inflammatory disease (PID), referred myalgia, etc.

2) The intensity of pain. Pain is assessed on an analogue scale from 0 to 10 (the worst pain ever experienced), reporting it in the chart with the numerical indications of intensity, for the points of greatest pain. This allows monitoring the algic sensitivity trend over time.

3) When you feel pain. If at the moment of penetration (the causes of introital pain mentioned earlier), during penetration (levator myalgia) or complete penetration (also check deep causes of dyspareunia and arousal quality).

4) How long does the pain last? If only during coitus or even after intercourse, up to two, three days or more. Symptom that, together with the introital site of pain, immediately suggests the presence of vulvar vestibulitis.

5) The associated symptoms are as follows:

a) Urinary (from the need to urinate after intercourse to urethral or cystic symptoms).
b) Intolerance to friction on clothes or manual stimulation during petting.
c) Intolerance to the insertion of a tampon for menstrual protection.
d) Occurrence of pain with the same characteristics as dyspareunia during the gynaecological examination that is therefore a valuable diagnostic tool for the majority of clients.

The physical examination, aimed at recognising the 'pain map' by quantifying the intensity of the pain at each point, allows completing the diagnosis and defining the aetiology, prognosis and diagnosis of the genital-pelvic pain disorder. Some medical causes may be responsible, at least partially, for the pain: the consequences of surgery, childbirth or the episiotomy in childbirth, endometriosis, vaginal or urethral infections, especially if recurrent, vaginal atrophy after menopause, oestrogen deficiency during the lactation period, the use of certain antidepressant and antipsychotic drugs (D'Ario, 2015).

If there do not seem to be physical causes that justify the pain, then the possible presence of psychological factors must be considered.

The first question to ask in order to evaluate the possible psychological element of the disorder is whether the pain is always there or in some circumstances. In our clinical practice, we have multidisciplinary teams to deal with this problem to consider the different aspects of pain: neurological, muscular, emotional and relational. In diagnostic examinations, pain must be taken into account as the central point of the disorder. In addition, any psychosexual conflict, personal distress and difficult relationships can be considered possible causes or contributory causes of pain, or conversely, pain can lead to conflicts and a refusal of sexual activity.

During the gynaecological examination, the woman should be asked to give an accurate description of the pain: when and where exactly she feels the pain, whether vulvar or vaginal, whether deep or superficial, whether a series of these. It is also good to investigate the quality of the pain, i.e. whether it is a burning sensation, acute or dull. For this purpose, a list of pain descriptors has been created so the client can describe it precisely (Melzack and Katz, 1992). It is also important to know what causes pain, in addition to coitus, and know how long it lasts. It is also recommended to ask for a description of the situation and activity, thoughts and feelings before, during and after pain and how the partner reacts to it. It is also important to ascertain the meaning of the pain; many women have a theory on why they feel pain during intercourse, and this can be helpful in resolving the symptom. It seems clear that pain during intercourse can lead to a reduction of arousal and lubrication, but the reduction in lubrication is not always considered the cause of genital-pelvic pain disorder and penetration.

Among the psychosocial factors involved, anxiety and depression are as strongly correlated with pain syndromes as much as problems are related to the relationship. *Relational causes* can contribute to the persistence and worsening of the perception of pain and to the worsening of the symptom:

- Lack of emotional intimacy.
- Conflicting relationships resulting in physical and emotional tension.
- Resistance to relationships in disappointing emotional contexts.
- Sexual problems of the partner, including anatomical problems, like congenital or acquired *recurvatum*.

Women experiencing severe pelvic or vulvar-vaginal pain during penetration are intolerant to vaginal penetration, but some of them may feel aroused, lubricated and experience orgasm with oral or manual stimulation. In fact, some virgin wives and their partners sometimes report a satisfactory sexual repertoire that, among other things, allows that the couple to postpone the request for help in time. When women have this symptom, they sometimes experience an involuntary contraction of the pelvic muscles even just by thinking they are going to be penetrated. Anxiety increases and penetration becomes impossible even using the smallest speculum. Many of these women have never had a gynaecological examination or used tampons. Women, in most cases, start therapy when their partner threatens divorce or when there is a desire to conceive a child.

The clinical experience invites focusing on the partner's role in the couple with this type of sexual dysfunction. The many years that generally go by from the onset of the symptom to the request for specific counselling make one reflect on a kind of complicity that is established in the couple's relationship. Several studies have in fact noticed some psychological characteristics in the partner of the woman with this disorder. The man is generally not very interested in sexuality, 'harmless', in the sense that he does not question the partner's symptom through demands, and he often has a sexual difficulty (erectile disorder or premature ejaculation) that is hidden by the woman's symptom.

In cases where penetration is impossible, the term white or unconsummated marriage is used, where attention is shifted to the couple especially in view of sexual treatment. Of particular importance is the framing of the possible collusion of the couple in the maintenance of the symptom, the analysis of possible secondary benefits from the symptom and the psycho-emotional support for both partners when approaching the most delicate phase of the therapy – full sexual intercourse (Kaplan, 1982). This phase requires experience, sensitivity and empathy for the therapist. It is important in these cases to examine the thoughts and emotions of these women and the meaning of the symptom. The scope is to offer an alternative to dysfunctional body language, rather than a simple vaginal access for penetration. As already mentioned, the partner must also be carefully evaluated and involved in the therapy.

Usually, the outcome is positive with motivated couples with good relationships, but there are difficulties in cases where there is panic, low motivation, relationship conflicts and uncooperative and unmotivated partners (Leiblum and Rosen, 2000).

2.2.5   *Final considerations on female sexual disorders*

The basic assumption shared by researchers is to try to explain the differences through a multidisciplinary approach that considers the complexity of the sexual response and the mutual interaction between organic and psychosocial factors. When the aetiological complexity of female sexual disorders can be correctly directed and a multifactorial and multisystemic diagnosis can be made, the therapy can be articulated, paying attention to modifying and treating the multiple biological, psychosexual and relational factors that contribute to the genesis of female sexual disorders. Several questionnaires are offered in addition to the physiological investigation tools to help investigate the female sexual response better.

Female sexual problems should be considered from an integrated perspective. Theory, research and sexual activity should be focused on meaning and function, taking into account both biological and psychological aspects. An integrated model is based on the collaboration between different professional figures for which the fundamental problem is related to understanding what defines a sexual dysfunction. The ideal approach to female sexual dysfunction includes the collaboration and integration of different specialists dealing with women's health.

Although there are significant anatomical-functional similarities between male and female sexuality, there are still some differences from a psychological and sexual experience point of view that do not allow us to intervene on female sexual dysfunctions the same way we intervene on male sexual dysfunctions.

Despite the existence of organic disorders, psychosocial, emotional and/or relational factors are much more important in determining the onset and/or maintenance of a sexual disorder in women. The risk of sex-pharmacology, as defined by Tiefer (2001), is to perpetuate genital function as the primary, 'natural' sexual experience.

2.3   Male sexual disorders

2.3.1   Classification of male sexual dysfunctions

The incidence of male sexual dysfunctions is surely increasing. This progression can be justified by environmental conditions like the increased toxicity of the substances contained in the air we inhale, especially in metropolitan areas, and also by causes that are intrinsic to the habits of modern life. For example, new clinical studies are made on the incidence of 'stress' in clients with an erectile dysfunction.

In recent research, the data shows that sexual dysfunctions are a widespread disorder in the male population in general; it is clear that, within each dysfunction, the traceable oscillations are linked to distress and, therefore, to the subjective meaning that the dysfunction has in the life of the individual. As underlined by several authors, the line of demarcation to conceptualise and recognise these dysfunctions at a diagnostic level is distress, a factor that requires in-depth investigation by researchers and consideration by the diagnostic-statistical manuals for mental disorders.

Male sexual dysfunctions, according to *DSM-5*, are distinguished into hypoactive sexual desire disorder, erection disorder (erectile dysfunction) and ejaculation disorder (premature or delayed).

2.3.2   Male hypoactive sexual desire disorder

Hypoactive sexual desire disorder has been introduced again for men. In the *DSM-III-R*, it was called 'sexual desire inhibition', and in the *DMS-IV*, it was divided into 'hypoactive sexual desire' and 'sexual aversion disorder'; the latter was deleted from the *DSM-5*. The increased focus on male sexual desire has led to acknowledging the hypoactive sexual desire disorder (HSDD) as a diagnostic category in *DSM-5*, defining it as a persistent or recurrent insufficient (or absence) of sexual/erotic thoughts or fantasies and desire for sexual activity. It is interesting to note that this disorder, historically and culturally deemed as a female one, has now significantly increased among men (Knopf & Seiler, 1993).

The problem of low sexual desire in men has been largely neglected in epidemiological research, although it is frequent in clinical practice (Lewis and Fugl-Meyer,

2004). Starting from an accurate sexual history that allows differentiating the diagnosis, the possible existence of systemic and hormonal diseases that can alter the perception of sexual desire should be verified, ending with the serological evalua tion of the hypothalamic-pituitary-gonadal axis and, where indicated, of the thyroid function (Carani *et al.*, 2005). Chronic systemic diseases include chronic hepatopathies, kidney failure, serious blood diseases and neo-plastic diseases in general.

Currently, the interest in HSDD is increasing, especially regarding its causes and possible treatments. As far as the aetiological hypotheses are concerned, great attention has been given to the biological component, i.e. the hormonal one; in fact, hypogonadism is mentioned as the main cause of the male hypoactive sexual disorder. While the hormonal component has a very important role in the male sexual desire, it emerges from literature that it is necessary to consider the other components involved in the disorder's onset or maintenance as well, thus using a biopsychosocial approach. A low sexual desire can affect the other phases of the sexual response, causing difficulties; therefore, it may happen that requests for help for other sexual dysfunctions (erectile dysfunction, premature or delayed ejaculation) hide a disorder in the desire area that, if not investigated correctly, could stay hidden.

In fact, research on men has always attributed a predominant role to biological factors, drastically reducing the importance of the emotional sphere and everything related to it. Pedro Nobre and Pinto-Gouveia (2003) has recently proposed a new model for the study of male desire, which is not just on an immediate response to erotic stimuli mediated solely by the presence of hormones but also on the influence on perceived desire for numerous aspects (age, existence of medical or psychological problems, degree of couple satisfaction, existence of erroneous beliefs on sex and on the use of distracting thoughts during intercourse).

The particularly interesting result that emerges is the fundamental role played by both the cognitive and emotional dimension. In men with HSDD, there is a lack of erotic fantasies and the presence of negative thoughts such as performance concerns (on erection) and negative emotions like sadness and shame. The activation of negative thoughts and emotions during sex can lead to not paying attention to sexual stimuli and, consequently, not perceiving any desire or arousal.

2.3.3   Erectile disorder

Erectile dysfunction is a very common discomfort that affects the life of those suffering from it in various ways; it affects social relationships and, in general, the quality of life, often causing depression, anxiety and loss of self-esteem (Hafez and Hafez, 2005; Levine, 2000; Lombardo *et al.*, 2004; Rhoden and Morgentaler, 2003; Sehgal and Srivastava, 2003; Steggall and Gann, 2002; Zhang *et al.*, 2002).

In the sexual response cycle, this type of disorder manifests itself in the excitement phase, where the erectile disorder in the male is in the inability to achieve or maintain an adequate erection necessary for penetration and to complete the sexual act. *DSM-5 TR* indicates that the fundamental characteristic of erectile disorder is a persistent or recurrent inability to achieve or maintain an adequate erection throughout intercourse (Criterion A). The anomaly must cause significant interpersonal discomfort or difficulty (Criterion B). The dysfunction is not attributable to another Axis I disorder (except for another sexual dysfunction) and is not exclusively due to the direct physiological effects of a substance (including drugs) or a general medical condition (Criterion C).

The criteria for erectile dysfunction are similar to those of the last edition, except for the necessary symptom of the loss of rigidity and the presence of the symptom 75%–100% of the time.

Epidemiological studies have shown the presence of various psychosocial factors involved in erectile disorders, such as depression, low self-esteem, anxiety and stress (Aydin et al., 2001). The aetiology of exclusively psychogenic erection disorders can be anyhow found in 40% of cases of erection disorders (Melnik and Abdo, 2005). Besides, the level of stress, the presence of depressive symptoms and, more generally, a poor mental health can negatively influence the erectile response. On the other hand, in terms of mainly physiological factors, cardio-circulation dysfunctions (Jackson et al., 2002; Kirby et al., 2005), diabetes mellitus (Klein et al., 2005; Fedele et al., 2001), high cholesterol levels (Seidman and Roose, 2000), neurological (Lue, 2001) and endocrinological diseases and HIV/AIDS (Dinsmore, 2005) can affect the erectile dysfunction. When cardiovascular disease, prostate disease, diabetes, ulcer, depression or oral problems can be excluded for the onset of erectile dysfunction, the presence of factors related to age and smoking or serious or moderate bladder problems have been detected (Nicolosi et al., 2003; Pourmand et al., 2004).

The pharmacological novelties marketed in recent years for the treatment of erectile dysfunction have prompted many men towards asking to be prescribed the 'miracle pill', but the rate of abandoning the drug and the need for clarification for many clients have led to continued efforts to help men and couples to a reappropriation of a sex life through an integrated psychological and pharmacological experience, where you can investigate the deeper and more symbolic meanings of male sexuality, the dynamics of the couple's relationship, real or imaginary, and sexual satisfaction in the broadest sense. In this perspective, the psychosomatic unity of man is not out of focus and the symptoms and pathological phenomena are investigated from a psychological and physiological point of view in a complementary way (Simonelli, 2006).

Clinical tradition has always stressed that the aetiology of the erectile disorder can be due to *psychological factors*, when the psychic elements are a primary factor in the onset and maintenance of the symptom. This type of disorder can be determined by immediate or situational causes like performance anxiety and events in the subject's recent history and by factors that affected the subject's development during childhood and adoption (Rosen, 2001; Bodie et al., 2003). Erectile dysfunction may be due to *combined factors* when it can be reasonably assumed that a general medical condition or the abuse of certain substances could have contributed to the emergence of the dysfunction, but they cannot be considered the only cause. Furthermore, the dysfunction may be due to a *general medical condition*, if it is considered enough to justify the onset and maintenance of the symptom. Medical causes can include, for example, diabetes mellitus, kidney failure, multiple sclerosis, etc. Finally, the disorder can be induced by the use of *substances*, when the erectile difficulties are caused by the use of drugs or particular classes of drugs like antidepressants, antihypertensives or neuroleptics (Simonelli, 2006).

Some authors (Althof, 2000; Sachs, 2003) believe that for the erectile dysfunction, the hasty attribution to organic or psychological factors should be rejected, embracing instead a more complex biopsychosocial model in which emotional, physical or physiological factors interact synergistically. In this sense, we have reached the need for a mainly organic or psychological diagnostic formulation.

For the *primary* erectile disorder, generally more serious from the prognostic point of view, it is necessary to ascertain if there are traumatic episodes associated with an immature psychological system or a negative orientation, with the presence of false beliefs related to intercourse. The dysfunction, in this case, would seem to be caused more by environmental influences.

For the *secondary* erectile disorder, it is necessary to verify any stressful situations that may have facilitated the onset of the symptom: asking the client whether there have been negative, but also positive, emotional episodes in the year before the onset of the disorder generally helps highlighting one or more thematic traces useful for the understanding and re-elaboration of the symptom. Sometimes a physiological episode of a lack of erection in a man's life can start the self-determining prophecy mechanism. The fear of a new failure creates a performance anxiety that inhibits the subsequent sexual response. Bonierbale *et al.* (2006) identified vulnerability factors consisting in beliefs that become fears in the relationship, negative beliefs on self-esteem, beliefs on sexuality in general, sexual relationships and the possible needs that the client attributes to himself, beliefs on the partner and adaption consequences resulting from the attempt to overcome the problem with personal strategies that are often inappropriate if not worsening.

The integrated model may require that the doctor and sexologist work together for the administration of pharmacology that, by limiting the urgency of the symptom, allows working on the more merging dynamics. An indication for this type of intervention requires a good evaluation of the client's personality in order to avoid a slow-down reaction from the drug and have a positive and collaborative attitude of the partner (Simonelli, 2006). In formulating a correct diagnosis, it is also fundamental to investigate causal factors related to the relationship. In fact, considering that the dysfunction is a problem for the couple and not just for the man, it is necessary to treat both partners where possible (Masters and Johnson, 1970; Crowe *et al.*, 1981; Hawton, 1985; Munoz, 1991; Althof, 2000). When the performance anxiety increases due to pressure by the partner, it often becomes the immediate cause of erectile dysfunction, simply because it is physiologically impossible for a man to maintain an erection when his body produces excessive amounts of norepinephrine due to anxiety. An early request for help means being able to count on the couple's resources to deal with the problem presented.

Recent research shows that, in most cases, the male disorder affects female sexuality negatively (Cayan *et al.*, 2004; Chevret *et al.*, 2004), leading to a mixed relational diagnosis in these cases. However, we must remember that the presence of the partner is useful not only in the treatment but also, and above all, in the diagnostic evaluation because her presence helps reconstruct the emotional context within which the symptom developed in a more complete way (Simonelli, 2006).

2.3.4 Premature ejaculation

Usually, ejaculation and orgasm occur simultaneously within the final phase of the sexual response cycle, but sometimes, they can occur independently of each other since they are two distinct phenomena. For example, ejaculation can take place without orgasm, or there may be an orgasm without ejaculation. While in animals, coitus is generally fast because this reduces their vulnerability and danger linked to predation, in the human species, it has a value linked not only to mating but also to the search for pleasure, which in itself is subjective and requires a certain voluntary and conscious control. In fact, orgasm is partly under the control of the ortho-sympathetic autonomic nervous system (ANS) and partly under the control of the voluntary nervous system (VNS). The sympathetic ANS regulates vasoconstriction and, particularly in humans, the contraction of the sperm pathway muscles, while the VNS regulates the possibility of conscious control of orgasm times. Usually, most young males learn by experience and age to delay orgasm, learning to recognise and manage the orgasmic inevitability point. In premature ejaculation, there is a difficulty in voluntary control so that the subject ejaculates earlier than he or she wishes. Shortly before, they generally experience the feeling of not being able to contain the intense excitement, and for this reason, they set up typical mechanisms to avoid non-control like thinking about other things, distracting themselves, avoiding foreplay and so on. However, in doing so, the perception of sensory afferences is enhanced, thus accelerating the automatic triggering of the orgasmic reflex. Today, pre-ejaculation is one of the most common forms of male sexual dysfunction. Various classifications, from the world of psychiatry to the world of urology, agree that early ejaculation is an ejaculation that occurs before or just after penetration, but before the client wishes and that it causes marked uneasiness to the subject and his or her partner. According to *DSM-5 TR*, premature ejaculation consists of 'persistent or recurrent ejaculation with minimal sexual stimulation before, on or shortly after penetration and before the person wishes it'. In the *DSM-5 TR*, compared to previous classifications, the criteria for premature ejaculation remained the same, except that premature ejaculation is such if it occurs within one minute after penetration into the vagina. For premature ejaculation in ratios other than vaginal ejaculation, no time criterion is indicated. Premature ejaculation must be distinguished into primary and secondary ejaculation from both an etiopathogenetic and clinical point of view for a regular approach to the problem. In this sense, it is necessary to recognise that the etiopathogenesis of premature ejaculation has a possible somatic and/or neurobiological nature that is often influenced by a significant psychological and interpersonal disorder component.

The temporal criterion is not a detail: if the dysfunction does not occur for a prolonged period of at least six months, it cannot be declared as such and can instead be read as a transient and transitory phenomenon, perhaps linked to periods of particular stress. What is most characteristic of this dysfunction is the lack of control on the ejaculatory process by the person, and it often occurs taking the person by surprise (Rowland, 2005). The many different definitions of premature ejaculation found in the literature make it very difficult to provide precise data on the prevalence of this sexual disorder, which is described as the most frequent in the male population. Overall, it is estimated that the prevalence of premature ejaculation can affect between 3% and 30% of the male population.

The results of a major international study (Laumann et al., 2005) showed a prevalence of premature ejaculation of 21%. Some recent researches that have tested very young men (18–25 years old) report a very high incidence of premature ejaculation that increases as age decreases, settling between 50% and 75% (Jannini and Lenzi, 2005). In fact, age, or rather, sexual inexperience, conditions the ability of ejaculatory control (Hartmann et al., 2005).

The causes of premature ejaculation are many and can be divided into organic and psychological; this is a simplistic distinction of the problem, considering the more frequent coexistence of both factors, which can strengthen each other. Each client should undergo a careful anamnestic evaluation followed by an accurate examination (genital, prostate) and the investigation of the case (haematochemical, hormonal, instrumental and neurophysiological tests, if required) (Jannini et al., 2002a, 2002b, 2011). Among the organic causes of premature ejaculation, the brevity of the frenulum is an important factor given the possibility of determining an increased penile sensitivity, predisposing to the ejaculatory problem at issue. In these cases, the surgical resolution of the problem is successful (Simonelli, 2006). Another possible organic element of the ejaculatory disorder is due to genital phlogosis for local hyperaemia and oedema: the examination of the semen and its treatment with a targeted antibiotic therapy can contribute to an improvement of the situation (Kamischke and Nieschlag, 2002). Neurological causes are many and are rarely of central origin (multiple sclerosis, spinal tumours, etc.) or more frequently peripheral (diabetic neuropathy, etc.) (Webster, 1994; Nusbaum et al., 2003). Finally, a further organic cause can be represented by a situation of hyperthyroidism, easily diagnosed through the plasma evaluation of thyroid hormones (Schuster and Ohl, 2002).

When possible, the therapy for premature ejaculation on an organic basis should be an aetiology therapy aiming at resolving the cause highlighted by the tests carried out (Montague et al., 2004). As far as pharmacological therapy is concerned, the most widely used therapy comprises selective serotonin reuptake inhibitors. Among these, the most commonly used drugs are fluoxetine, sertraline and paroxetine, to be taken as a chronic therapy with different efficacy profiles and possible indication of undesirable effects (Kim and Seo, 1998; Waldinger et al., 2005; Rosen et al., 1999). A further therapeutic possibility is based on the use of topical remedies to reduce penile sensitivity (retardant condoms, anaesthetic ointments, etc.) (Busato and Galindo, 2004).

There are numerous psychological factors that can potentially interfere with a man's sexual health and could worsen or support a premature ejaculation condition. In this context, it is possible to distinguish factors related to the person's sexual history (like, among others, the sexual education received and any sexual abuse suffered), individual factors (physical appearance, mood deflection or clear depression, performance anxiety, alexithymia), as well as factors related to the person's relational ability. However, several authors agree in identifying a certain difficulty of interpersonal relationships for the person (Symonds *et al.*, 2003; Althof, 2010).

According to psychoanalytic theories, the person suffering from this disorder experiences a fundamental ambivalence towards women, characterised by intense, albeit unconscious, hostile and punitive feelings and by the conscious desire for a relationship. The person's emotional immaturity makes him incapable of facing the ambivalence that is expressed by means of symptoms through which the man prevents his partner from fully enjoying sexual intercourse (Simonelli, 2006; Dèttore, 2001). Marital disorders (such as a rejection of the partner, hostility and power struggles within the couple) often condition sexual activity in a negative way (Athanasiadis, 1998; Metz and Pryor, 2000). The involvement of both partners in the therapeutic process is often very functional for the couple in order to find or develop new ways of experiencing sexuality in the light of shared and mutual pleasure.

What maintains the disorder may seem a paradox: not being able to regulate the increasing intensity of arousal, the man could try, to avoid premature ejaculation, distracting himself to 'not feel'. However, the less he pays attention to sensory sensations, the less he has the chance to learn to recognise the physical sensations before the point of orgasmic inevitability, so he is unable to develop the physiological control ability for the ejaculatory reflex. The partner may have an angry and frustrated reaction, developing feelings due to a lack of attention by the partner, or may unconsciously become rejecting or punishing. What often happens is that the couple is no longer available to search pleasure together but develops an idea of sexuality more in terms of a performance to demonstrate something to the other. In addition, the resulting dissatisfaction that is generated in both partners can lead to conflicts, communication rejection and an emotionality characterised by anxiety and/or anger, and this can also affect the desire and arousal sexual response.

Anxiety also plays an important role in expressing the symptom and is very often linked to one's experience of pleasure (Rowland *et al.*, 2010). Usually, an anxiety associated with pleasure generates a perceptive defence mechanism against excitement, so the man begins to pay attention to the outside rather than to the inside of the body (Simonelli, 2006). The man then could become a spectator of sexual intercourse, losing contact with his erotic perceptions and the premonitory sensations of ejaculation (Kaplan, 1974, 1979; Zilbergeld, 1992).

Lastly, premature ejaculation could also be a sexual symptom secondary to another disorder; for example, it could be a difficulty of the erection, or it may be the response to a sexual dysfunction of the partner (Simonelli, 2006). The most used behavioural therapies are squeeze and the stop-and-start therapy, both oriented towards the acquisition of greater control over average levels of arousal. Through specific exercises, the person is able to gain greater control over ejaculation times and recover self-esteem that translates in greater confidence during sexual intercourse and a reduced anxiety. On its own, this process is able to extend ejaculation times, as well as allowing the client to experience greater freedom and a variety of sexual approaches. Kegel exercises applied to the male pelvic muscle are also very useful for more body awareness and to relax the pelvic area of the coccyges muscle especially before penetration (Metz and Pryor, 2000).

The scope of integrating medical therapy with a mental/educational approach is to optimise the treatment's result, helping the client regain control of ejaculation in a stable way (Althof, 2010). The therapy should include not only the client's awareness of the pre-ejaculatory sensations to manage the ejaculatory reflex but also the analysis of anxiety in entering into a relationship, enhancing the client's resources and ability to get involved and facilitating the possibility of establishing an intimate relationship (Simonelli, 2006).

In this sense, it can be extremely useful to involve the partner in the diagnostic and therapeutic process permanently because the recovery of a greater complicity in a sexual relationship guarantees a further stimulus for the client to recover his self-esteem and sense of masculinity and adequacy in the management of his sexuality.

2.3.5   Delayed ejaculation

According to the DSM-5, to talk about delayed ejaculation, the individual must report, in all or almost all (about 75%–100%) sexual intercourses and without the delay being intentional, a marked delay in ejaculation and a marked infrequency or absence of ejaculation. Attention should be paid to the differentiation of diagnosis with other medical conditions (peripheral neuropathies, prostate disease, etc.) or similar substance-induced disorders.

The severity of delayed ejaculation varies considerably from client to client and ranges from a completely involuntary and occasional inhibition of the ejaculation to such a severity meaning that the client has never experienced an orgasm in the company of a partner. The lightest form, often not submitted to clinicians, is the one characterised by the inhibition of the ejaculatory reflex in anxiety situations. Anxiety can be related to where the coitus takes place, the woman with whom sexual activity is shared, the extent of guilt, inadequacy, censorship of pleasure and much more.

The most common situation is characterised by a global and generalised inhibition, and the man is unable to reach pleasure with his partner. Delayed ejaculation can be primary and secondary. Primary ejaculation is characterised by a correlated absence of orgasmic response from the very first sexual experiences: clients belonging to this category only reach 'extra-coitus' orgasms and never in a vaginal sphere. In the case of secondary delayed ejaculation, the client develops this dysfunction after an initial sexual health and well-being, often in association with a traumatic experience, a woman with particular psychophysical characteristics or conflictual and/or blackmail couple dynamics. The prognosis is certainly more favourable in the latter case.

The pathophysiological mechanisms underlying delayed ejaculation can be of a psychogenic, organic and iatrogenic nature (drug or surgical). In first place among the organic causes at the base of this disorder is the neurological ones represented by the following: marrow cancer or traumas, multiple sclerosis, sensitive neuropathies (e.g. diabetic) and surgical lesions of the nervous system (Simonelli, 2006). From an organic point of view, even the normal hormonal structure participates in the physiology of the ejaculatory reflex. The reduction of androgenic levels or the reduced sensitivity to them is considered a determining factor in this proposition, resulting, for example, in a situation of hyperprolactinemia, induced by drugs or pituitary pathology (Romanelli *et al.*, 2000). The drugs potentially able to interfere with the ejaculatory reflex, delaying it, are antihypertensives with a central action, methyldopa and clonidine. An attentive diagnostic procedure is essential to set up a correct therapeutic strategy.

As far as organic-based forms are concerned, the frequent occurrence of degenerative or secondary neurological pathologies to lesions of the innervation pathways leaves poor results at every therapeutic attempt. The psychogenic forms must be tackled in a personalised way, with a psychotherapeutic approach that must involve not only the client but also his partner in order to restore a normal interaction within the couple (Simonelli, 2006). Despite a wide variability from subject to subject, it is possible to affirm that in the elderly male, there is an extension of the arousal phase with a delayed achievement of an adequate erectile response. This is followed by an extension of the *plateau* phase (time from the erection to ejaculation) to delineate a situation of delayed ejaculation that occurs with a reduction of the propulsive force upon expulsion. Despite the possible qualitative and quantitative modifications that the sexual activity of the elderly man can undergo, it is interesting to mention the possibility of a maintained sexuality for a large percentage of subjects belonging to this category (Helgason *et al.*, 1996).

Historically, several explanations have been offered as possible causes for the delayed ejaculation, but the psychoanalytic literature seems to agree on some points: the presence of a retained aggressiveness, the unconscious will to punish the woman by not sharing pleasure with her and the fear of conceiving and of the responsibility that would result (Friedman, 1973) from this. In the context of their studies, Masters and Johnson (1970) traced the causes of delayed ejaculation back to a repressive religious education with heavy feelings of guilt towards sex and one's own sexuality. In the clinical experience with these people, it is quite common to notice overly invasive and controlling female figures in providing care. Therefore, the presence of a significant female figure is dangerous, and the tension that can arise from intimacy and relational demands is very often expressed through feelings of anger or emotional closure.

Always within childhood experiences, it is frequent to have excessive expectations by the parents in the education received, so strong as to inhibit different forms of free expression. Excessive control prevents man from living the sensations coming from the body and consequently from letting go towards the orgasmic experience (Simonelli, 2006). Regardless of the cause, the worry for the ejaculation diminishes the excitement, leading to an obsessive self-observation that blocks pleasure (Waldinger and Schweitzer, 2005); instead, during masturbation, the subject is generally free from this control, and as he can rely on erotic fantasies, he has less chance of the symptom occurring (Lo Piccolo, 1985). In these cases, it is good to investigate, with respect to the specific symptom, how it is expressed, and then after having identified whether it is primary or secondary, a situational or generalised disorder, the therapist will have to understand if the difficulty in ejaculating appears only during intercourse or if it occurs while masturbating as well. The aim of sexual therapy is, on the one hand, to investigate the fears that may be associated with the ejaculatory event and the sexual act (fear of pregnancy, sexually transmitted diseases, abortion, loss of control) and, on the other hand, to help the person conceive sexuality as a moment of pleasure for himself, with the intention of restoring a balance between the erotic and inhibiting potential (Simonelli, 2006). The collaboration with the partner is decisive to build this new dimension of pleasure together, and the partners must create a relaxing atmosphere that facilitates the expression of erotic sensations and, consequently, decrease the attention and expectations on the purpose of the encounter. For this reason, the couple will be asked to focus their attention on pleasure rather than on the result of the performance. Vice versa, negative feelings of hostility, emotional distance, detachment, lack of pleasure or disgust may also emerge. In these cases, it is good to emphasise them and make them express themselves openly rather than letting them manifest themselves in sexuality (Simonelli, 2006). In some cases, it could be useful to associate psychological therapy with a pharmacological therapy. Several studies have shown that the serotonergic system has an inhibitory role in ejaculation, while the dopaminergic system can facilitate it; therefore, dopaminergic or anti-serotonergic drugs facilitate the ejaculatory process and can be integrated in sexual therapy (Perelman, 2006; Nurnberg et al., 2003).

2.3.6   Traumatic aspects related to male organic pathology

Much has been said in recent years on the importance of andrological prevention in young people from ages 14 to 20. Anomalies and pathologies of the genital system in adolescents and young adults are often diagnosed late for historical and cultural reasons. Moreover, the problem related to a diagnostic delay has worsened in Italy because of the abolition of the obligatory military service that was when young men underwent a medical examination that involved the genitals too. The presence of a psychologist is fundamental both in the pre-operative and post-operative phases.

In the pre-surgery phase, the clinician can evaluate the client's personality and underline the impact that surgery may have on his psychic balance, as well as investigate the motivation and expectations of the individual and couple. It must be considered that for surgery to be successful, the expectations of the partner are as relevant as those of the clients. Besides, psychotherapy is very useful to prepare the couple for the post-surgical adaptation, providing comprehensive explanations on the risks and possible complications. During the post-surgery period, the psychological work should deal with the adaptation, acceptability and satisfaction deriving from surgery. The importance of psychotherapy for sexual dysfunctions of organic origin is often underestimated, forgetting that surgery pertaining to sexuality should respect a somatopsychic as well as psychosomatic approach and that the treatment should be directed to returning a satisfactory sexual life to the client, not just a rigid and functional erection. In fact, in urological practice, clear biological problems often have different outcomes depending on the history of the client or couple facing a defined symptom or surgery. The main anomalies of organic origin are described later.

Phimosis

Phimosis is the most frequent pathology of the male genitals and consists in the inability to retract the foreskin due to a congenital or acquired foreskin shrinkage (secondary to multiple inflammations: balanoposthitis). This situation prevents the client not only from masturbating with the unexposed glans but also causes discomfort if not pain and difficulty during coitus due to the abnormal contact of the penis with the vagina. It is solved surgically under local anaesthesia in an outpatient's clinic, with so-called circumcision.

Congenital penile curvature

Congenital penile curvature (*recurvatum penis*) is believed to be due to a disharmonious development of the penis tissues (cavernous bodies and/or spongy body) during the first years of life. It may vary for different curvature severity and directions: most often, the deviation is ventral (towards the abdomen) and sometimes lateral (more frequently to the left). Disorders pertaining to the congenital penile curvature mainly vary depending on the curvature angle. Usually, it does not cause pain in the erection and already exists in the prepubescence, although the problem is clearer with physical growth.

Induratio penis plastica

Induratio penis plastica (IPP) is an andrological pathology of which many aspects still need to be clarified. IPP is characterised by the formation of a fibrotic plaque on the tunica albuginea of the penis that limits penile elasticity during erection causing a curvature towards the diseased side, pain and, in some cases, erectile dysfunction. Depending on the client's stage, there are different therapeutic alternatives, both pharmacological and surgical.

Therefore, we are talking about a 'purely' organic pathology that can be cured with 'purely' medical treatments that restore the client's penile function. Even if IPP is an organic disease that can be treated both pharmacologically and surgically, it could affect the sexual and relational life; it is, therefore, very important that the doctor work alongside the psycho-sexologist from the very first moment. In fact, the few studies on the matter highlight the consequences of this pathology on an emotional and relational level.

At the time of diagnosis, the person is confronted with a condition he never would have imagined to experience: suffering from an 'unknown' pathology that jeopardises the ability to undertake a coital relationship. *Induratio plastic penis*, in addition to affecting the male genital organ, affects the male identity; just think about the importance of the penis for the man, its size, its shape and its perfect functionality, adding the sociocultural factor for which a man's body image rotates around the phallus. In fact, it emerges that due to the deformity of the penis, the person with *induratio penis plastica* tends to describe himself as 'abnormal', 'disgusting' and, even, as a 'half man'. The resulting level of distress could also lead to the development of serious illnesses like depression.

As we can imagine, this could have a negative impact on the person's sexual functioning. Research in literature shows that the man feels less masculine, no longer attractive and worried about not being able to satisfy his partner as he used to. Especially because of pain, clients often experience a strong performance anxiety leading them to experience a decrease in desire; in fact, they often prefer avoiding intercourse and generally avoiding any kind of intimacy, believing that their sexual life has come to an end. What happens then in a couple's life? Research shows that IPP can have emotional consequences not only for the individual but also for the partner. The devaluation of oneself, giving up on sexuality and the resulting anxiety-depressive disorder in the man frequently has repercussions, so he develops, if the plaque formation hypothesis is linked to the micro-trauma caused by sexual intercourse, guilt or anger.

It also emerges that the partner often has difficulty in accepting the pathology and the client often has difficulty and embarrassment talking to her about his worries. It must be considered that these studies have been conducted on heterosexual couples. There is a lack of studies in literature investigating the experience of a homosexual couple even if some clinical experiences seem to show that the negative effects are amplified both by having a partner without a penile deformity that always reminds the person of his deformity and by social stigmatisation. Psychotherapy can be very useful for helping the person accept the changes due to the pathology and for encouraging and enhancing the use of sexual practices alternative to coitus so that the couple can develop a different idea on sexuality, no longer one of performance but of being playful and emotional.

It is, therefore, very important that all medical treatments be accompanied by psychosexual counselling; this is very useful in favouring the transition from past regrets to confidence in the pharmacological or surgical treatment that are very helpful to the therapy. This is even more true in cases of surgical treatments where the already complex clinical situation of the IPP is also aggravated by the thera-peutic options given to the person that often mean a shortening of the shaft or an altered penile form.

2.3.7 What we can do

What measures must be taken to improve the health of the modern male population? The way of thinking has a negative effect on the sexual response and modulates mood and anxiety effects. Cultural, religious, social, educational and family status are all determinants of the sexual response. The basis for empathy towards young clients is to understand the source of their discomfort because unwanted thoughts can be changed by identifying and challenging it. Helping to overcome such wor-ries (even the most trivial ones may disregard more serious illnesses), by providing all the necessary information, proves to be a very useful educational path.

Men should be urged to follow a healthier lifestyle in terms of diet, body and behaviour. The classic belief about male success in youth is that 'high self-esteem is achieved through sexual performance and social success, and this increases the charm of a relationship with women'. It now seems that the sexuality of the new millennium is directed towards what we seem or want to be and that removes us from the interpersonal and social relationships that are at the basis of a shared experience for a man and a woman. From public information campaigns, preven-tion weeks, American-style 'talk-shows', it emerges clearly that men tend to hide health issues more than women.

There is still so much to be done to prove the effectiveness of prevention strate-gies in prospective randomised trials with control groups, but it is also true that if male public prevention is not organised, we will never have concrete answers.

Chapter 3

Male genitalia

Psychosexual aspects

Paolo Maria Michetti and Giovanni Simonelli

3.1 Introduction[1]

When entering the field of sexology, the concept of 'normality' is not reliable. Those parameters that seem well defined in traditional medicine are faded here, and sometimes it is also dangerous to try to define them because of the risk of turning men with traits of insecurity, anxiety or immaturity into 'sick' persons. So morphological characteristics, measurements (e.g. genital size), quality (of erection according to the rigidity or ejaculatory impulse) and timing (of intercourse, reaching orgasm, etc.) are absolute variables that must not be coded too rigidly, especially if they do not cause discomfort and do not remove satisfaction from the person or couple.

Recently, the concept of 'sexual discomfort' is gaining ground in the field of sexual medicine, understood as an anatomical-functional characterisation, a symptom or type of behaviour that does not divert greatly from the majority but is a source of insecurity and suffering. It is the task of every andrologist to be able to accept this discomfort, on the one hand, with effective and, if possible, resolutive counselling and, on the other, if possible, avoiding medicalisation and the transformation into a pathology. The salient topics for the request for tests related to the morpho-functional aspects of male genitals concerns congenital anomalies and the results of their surgery, genital pain or fear of pain and penile dysmorphic disorder.

3.2 Congenital abnormalities of the penis and surgical outcomes

A positive medical history for surgery in the genital region is deemed as a possible disruptive factor with regard to the approach to normal sexual activity.

Circumcision is a procedure described since ancient times and is one of the most common surgeries performed in the world; however, there is still much debate on its real effect on male sexuality. Few studies have addressed the effects of circumcision performed during infancy to sexuality and the consequences of circumcision performed on adult men has received even less attention. One of the most widespread discernments regards the likely role of keratinisation of the glans that

DOI: 10.4324/9781003508670-4

could lead to a reduction in sensitivity, therefore, of sexual arousal. In the 1960s, Masters and Johnson (1966) excluded this condition with a study that showed no differences in the penile sensory perception between circumcised and uncircumcised men.

A very detailed study by Sorrels *et al.* (2007) compared sensitivity in 19 different penile areas between circumcised and uncircumcised subjects, stating that circumcision removes the most sensitive areas of the penis and decreases blood pressure sensitivity. Bleustein *et al.* (2005) conducted a comparative study between 36 circumcised and 43 uncircumcised clients using a series of somatic tests evaluating the vibratory, spatial, thermal and pressure function of nerve fibres of various calibres, finding no statistically important differences in the results of these tests between the two groups. Another number is the sample of Kigozi *et al.* (2008), who conducted a randomised trial on 4,456 clients (2,210 underwent circumcision in adulthood and 2,226 uncircumcised) with whom they investigated the relationship between circumcision and sexual function and satisfaction. Sexual desire, erection and ejaculation were evaluated with questionnaires. No statistically significant differences were reported between the two groups. Kim and Pang (2006) did not report any differences in arousal, erection and ejaculation between the two groups in their study of 373 sexually active men (255 adult circumcised and 158 non-circumcised); however, the circumcised clients showed a decrease in pleasure in masturbation and sexual intercourse.

In conclusion, it is difficult to make definitive statements on the effects of circumcision on sexuality. In our experience, circumcision solves a situation that is incompatible with a normal and satisfying sexual activity, and overall, the benefits outweigh the costs. It is clear that the indication must be correct, and the surgical technique must also take into account the aesthetic desires of the client as well as solving the preputial stenosis. A partial postectomy is certainly more accepted in terms of image and of preserved sensitivity for the client, but it exposes the client to the risk of complications like a much more frequent scarring.

The literature on frenuloplasty is even more scarce: only one work (Rajan *et al.*, 2006) in the last ten years reports a consistent series (209) of short frenulum cases treated with classical technique. The author reports a high satisfaction rate in clients that underwent surgery and without going into the detail of sexual satisfaction, which is supposed to have been good. Gallo *et al.* (2010) analyse the beneficial effects of frenulum plastic in a limited, non-randomised sample of subjects affected by premature ejaculation, with an average increase in intravaginal ejaculatory latency time (IELT) of 2.46 minutes.

In our experience, this kind of benefit is not univocal, and we deem that the increased genital sensitivity sometimes reported by subjects with premature ejaculation is not just for the frenulum but also extended to the balano-preputial furrow and to the glans in general. In the same way, clinical experience suggests that circumcision is not a valid average for premature ejaculation either, where the incidence rate of this disorder among the millions of circumcised men in the world is superimposable on that of non-circumcised men.

3.3　Male dyspareunia and fear of genital pain

When we talk about male genital pain, we must refer not only to what a man feels during sexual intercourse (Luzzi and Law, 2006) but also to the pain he is afraid of feeling and that conditions him in his approach to sex, causing an avoidance or the appearance of three dysfunctions: erectile dysfunction, premature ejaculation or delayed ejaculation. The term 'dyspareunia' is used in current nosology for both sexes.

Literature is copious only for what pertains the female side of the matter. Y. M. Binik (Binik, 2005; Binik *et al.*, 2000) has provided quality contributions on this topic in the last ten years and believes that the male version of dyspareunia is quite rare because of the very scarce scientific production on the matter. In our experience, genital pain or the fear of it greatly affects male sexuality, but these are often omitted, misunderstood by the client or not recognised by the doctor.

A very frequent picture is that of the hypersensitivity of the glans. Since the age of puberty development, the man avoids lowering the foreskin and coming into contact with the glans because of its great sensitivity. This sensitivity is maintained until it is easier to explore the mucosa (through a progressive keratinisation) and it becomes a source of pleasure rather than an intolerable discomfort. This condition can be confused with phimosis, but in this case, there is no real congenital or acquired stenosis of the preputial cylinder but rather, an elasticity connected to the 'dishabituation' of uncovering it. Sometimes, these men have a perfectly normal sexual activity; other times, they fear it, imagining the constriction in the vagina as an unbearable source of discomfort. The idea that the foreskin uncovers during penetration or in the condom is a source of serious concern and puts off the beginning of sexual activity. At other times, the fear is quite evident at the moment of penetration, when (due to the awareness of the feared hypersensitivity) the man loses the rigidity of the penis, making the sexual act impossible.

Another symptomatology resulting from this situation is that of extreme precociousness in sexual intercourse: the afferent genital stimulation during penetration is strongly increased by the fact that the glans is uncovered when the genital sensations are always mediated by the preputial cover. Lastly, less frequent but possible, and observed during my clinical experience, is the association with delayed ejaculation. Here, the genital sensations during penetration can be experienced as unpleasant, thus not leading, in a crescendo, to orgasm when masturbation makes one aware of the protected genital stimulation giving the desired result. In all these cases, a real re-education of genital sensitivity is indispensable: daily experiences of contact with the uncovered glans while practising hygiene or not, and also self-masturbation, better if using a lubricant like Vaseline or other oils, will allow overcoming the problem gradually.

Perhaps it is not known that at the origin of an unconsummated marriage, there is often the issue of fear of pain for the male. In a personal case study concerning a sample of eight unconsummated marriages in the last year and presented at the Congress in 2009 (Michetti *et al.*, 2009), 75% of men reported that they expected feeling pain during the act that was generally associated with a poor knowledge of male and female genital anatomy and physiology. More in general, sexual ignorance characterised this sample of men, more than 50% of whom reported that they had never seen explicit coital images; it is good to observe also that the level of education of this population consisted mainly in the achievement of a degree and more rarely that of a high school diploma.

3.4   Penile dysmorphophobia

It is not an infrequent phenomenon but probably an underestimated one: subjective suffering for a supposedly small penis that is not objectively so. Concerns on the size of one's own penis and the desire to have a larger one are frequent in the male population and cannot be defined as pathological. However, anxiety and concern on the size of the penis can sometimes reach such an intensity and quality that it is possible to deem them as pathological. Penile dysmorphophobia (Andreasen *et al.*, 1977), a morbid condition consisting in an anxiety-depressive syndrome in people that even if they are anatomically normal, they consider the appearance and size of their penis as unsuitable, inadequate. Even if the shaft is normal, the man perceives it as too small compared to the image he created for himself.

In most cases, this is an alteration in the perception of the body image. In fact, it is as if these people see their sexual organ through a deforming mirror; they are certain that they have a penis that is too small to have a relationship with their partner. Perceiving their body as deformed leads these people to developing a series of emotional and relational perturbations, as if enduring a real handicap; the condition leads to a clinically significant discomfort or to a high level of alteration of relations in society, work or other important areas. They attribute a direct link with the social respectability of which they feel deprived due to the size of their penis. Therefore, the sexual identity of the client could be altered because it is intrinsically linked to what the penis looks like, to the extent of making them feel 'real or complete men' (Cohen *et al.*, 2000).

Men tend to undergo continuous comparisons regarding the size of their genitals in changing rooms of gyms or sports centres, always paying attention to not exposing themselves to others to avoid being looked at and then mocked.

This disquiet due to the size of the penis can also upset the sexual partner because anxiety can be transmitted. After years of anxiety, these people first consult a doctor who, after reassuring the client on the 'normal' state of their penis, for example, by showing reference tables, is then asked to perform a surgical enlargement of the penis. The doctor, realising these clients' irrational beliefs, sends them to a psychosexologist or a psychiatrist for an evaluation of the dysmorphic symptom, trying to assign it to a precise psychopathology and treat it as such.

The treatment of a penis that is too small has created considerable difficulties so far. The first was due to the fact that effective surgical techniques to modify the size of the penis were not available until recently. Without a concrete urological/andrological response, the only words these clients often heard were 'your penis is of normal size'. The request of the client was, in this way, avoided because the objective register was used instead of listening to the individual suffering, to which no suited answers could be given. Collaboration with the psychologist or psycho-sexologist meant progress: the subjective dimension gained acknowledgment and, therefore, right to a cure. Psychosexual treatment is indicated for those clients whose request for intervention is based on the illusion that a larger penis protects them from the risk and compensates their inability to experience the dimension of intimacy of a relationship, which is something they desire but fear.

Then another type of client probably has narcissistic personality traits and a more limited relational capacity; therefore, these clients are more resistant to psychotherapeutic treatment. For them, the construction of a relationship with other men or women inevitably goes through interfacing a penis judged as normal. They do not tolerate the intimate dimension of a relationship and seem to have little interest in it. They diligently pursue a performance-oriented sexuality, and the relationship with the other is structured on the surface, a pursuit and display of external attributes: work role, beauty, development of body muscle mass, power, status-symbol objects and, 'if possible', a larger penis.

3.5   Varicocele

Varicocele is a pathology that affects the testicular vascular system, characterised by dilation and incontinence of the testicular (or spermatic) veins. It affects about 10%–20% of the general male population. It may already occur in preadolescent age (in 2%–2.5% of boys aging between 7 and 10 years of age), but the age at which it normally occurs is that of sexual maturation, between 11 and 16 years of age. It mainly affects the left testicle (95%) and rarely the right testicle (5%); this is due to the different anatomical characteristics between the two vascular pathways.

It is not yet clear why varicocele has a harmful effect on spermatogenesis only in a few men. It has been hypothesised that many pathophysiological mechanisms are at the basis of this phenomenon like hypoxia, hyperthermia, adrenal reflux, hormonal dysfunctions, autoimmunity, oxidative stress and apoptosis, partly due to the altered testicular venous drainage that occurs with varicocele. Usually, the diagnosis of varicocele takes place primarily during an andrological examination.

In most cases, there are no symptoms, but when it is symptomatic, there is a dull pain in one or both testicles, a feeling of heaviness or tension in the scrotum, palpable veins in the scrotum and felt discomfort in the testicle or on the affected side of the scrotum. The testicle on the side of the dilated veins is smaller (because of the lower blood flow). As said, varicocele can be detected through clinical examination, although a physical examination tends to underestimate the real incidence of this pathology.

With regards to the ultrasound, the objectives of the Doppler study of the pampiniform plexus are as follows: to demonstrate the presence of a pathological venous reflux, to classify the varicocele according to its endoscrotal extension, to distinguish the monolateral forms from the bilateral ones and to assess the state of gonads and epididymes, with particular attention to calculating the testicular volume and demonstrating the possible relapse of varicocele after surgery. Based on the findings obtained with the earlier procedures, we can obtain information on the presence or absence of varicocele and the extent and location of pathological venous refluxes.

Varicocele requires surgery and is based on anterograde or retrograde sclerotherapy, or on the retrograde embolisation of the venous vessels; the surgical approach can be either scrotal or inguinal, with microsurgery or laparoscopy techniques.

3.6   Psychoeducation on sexual problems in young people

The resolution of some minor sexual problems can be achieved through appropriate and specific sex education aimed at filling knowledge gaps or correcting erroneous and distorted views of one's own sexual physiology and anatomy, also due to age-related changes. Hence, it is paramount to disseminate proper knowledge of the male's sexual anatomy and physiology to clarify any doubts and drop excessive myths concerning the size of the penis.

Note

1 This chapter discusses the psychosomatic aspects of the male genitals in normal conditions and with a disease. The specialist text of the following paragraphs was written by Paolo Maria Michetti and Giovanni Simonelli of the Department of Urology at the University 'La Sapienza' in Rome.

Chapter 4

The correlation between trauma and sexual dysfunctions

Elena Isola

4.1 Trauma and its consequences

In our clinical experience, we often face issues in the sexual sphere, whose traumatic aetiology is prevalent.

The word 'trauma' comes from the Greek *traum'a*, and it means 'wound', 'laceration', 'damage' (Winnik, 1969) or 'shock'. This word was used for the first time to explain the psychological impact of stressful events by a German neurologist, who coined the term 'psychic trauma' (Eulenburg, 1978; van der Hart *et al.*, 1990). In clinical and scientific literature, the expression 'traumatic event' is quite common and the term 'trauma' is often used as a synonym (Kardiner and Spiegel, 1947). In the last two decades, many research projects have been carried out on the concept of trauma and its psychopathological effects: the related debate is getting more and more extensive to include new important discoveries that are positive for basic research and clinical practice and exert major effects at social level. Getting to know trauma, the effects on the person's functioning and the related disorders allows us to understand how important the safety relationship is to our clients. Please note first that the treatment of trauma-based sexual disorders demands even more caution if we consider that sexuality falls within the sphere of intimacy – both emotional and physical. Traumatic experiences – as we know – may be reactivated in the presence of any minimum stimulus, which may be 'considered' as dangerous, and they can activate the disturbed brain circuits by producing abnormal quantities of stress hormones. This makes the individual feel as if he/she were overwhelmed and flooded with unpleasant emotions, intense physical sensations and impulsive behaviours.

Clinicians need some therapeutic tools to tackle the client's moments of difficulty, which inevitably affect the therapeutic process by originating relational difficulties, deadlocks, impasses and, sometimes, an event therapy dropout. Bottom-up techniques coupled with sexual therapy strongly support the therapeutic work that may sometimes expose the client to unwanted re-traumatisation. For instance, let us think about the activation that sex therapy may cause in the process of treatment when the client starts following some indications involving intimacy and actions that are too much too early for him/her. The work on traumatic experiences

DOI: 10.4324/9781003508670-5

helps develop progressive awareness about the body's fundamental role: traumatic memories are not integrated into the person's own story; however, the experience is recorded in an implicit way at the level of body patterns. Therefore, traumatic experiences are not remembered, but they are re-experienced and cannot be controlled since they are not consciously integrated.

To process all the effects of a traumatic or painful experience, you must pay attention to the body so that you can modulate the activation without switching it off and without dissociating it from the somatic experience and access body memories, i.e. procedural memories.

The clients who have survived serious maltreatment are often not able to take appropriate care of themselves and talk about a sense of detachment from their own body, which is frequently used to find relief and solace from unbearable feelings and urges in the form of self-endangering behaviours, substance abuse, eating disorders and risky behaviours. The body with its different representations and functioning levels may become a tool to express several levels of meta-cognitive deficits, i.e. the expression of dissociative phenomena. A study is worth mentioning to the purpose (Farina *et al.*, 2011), whose goal was to assess somatoform and psychoform dissociation in clients with psychogenic female sexual dysfunctions like orgasmic disorder, dyspareunia and vaginism. A strong association was observed between somatoform disorders and psychogenic female sexual dysfunctions (FSDs), and outcomes are in line with the idea that some FSD forms could be considered as somatoform dissociative disorders following traumatic experiences.

Therefore, when the sexual disorder has a post-traumatic origin, using EMDR appears to be an effective and final treatment since it fosters the processing and integration of those traumatic experiences underlying the disorder that had been stored in a dysfunctional way in the client's memory networks.

4.2   Specific aspects of trauma, particularly in childhood

The word 'trauma' describes all threatening and overwhelming experiences that we have not been able to integrate. Sometimes, attachment figures are the very same source of threat, and this generates a conflict between the desire to ask them for protection and support and the need to protect oneself from them. Relational trauma can come from strangers, too, as for bullying, hate crimes, sexual violence and physical abuse. Some events, like accidents or natural disasters, are not caused by other people; however, they can be quite traumatising anyway. Trauma may be caused by a single event (for instance, an accident, rape, an experienced act of crime or a natural disaster) or by repeated events. Other traumatising events may include long-lasting or chronical situations (like serious abuse and neglect against children, war, deportation, concentration camps). When traumatising events occur repeatedly in the first years of life and they are caused by an attachment figure and/ or when no one is available to safely resort to, their effects and consequences may be difficult to solve in a natural way.

However, not all traumatic, highly stressful events originate a traumatic wound and the person's inability to recover naturally and in time. This depends first on the age when the traumatic event is experienced and, secondly, on the individual's psychophysical conditions when the traumatic experience occurs, which could possibly affect the potential resilience we all have within us. This is the reason why not all the people who experience a stressful event shall be traumatised. A person's level of traumatisation depends on two interacting factors, i.e. the objective and subjective characteristics of the event, which define the individual's psychic energy and mental efficiency that make up the integration capacity (van der Hart et al., 2006). Some events may be more traumatising than other ones, i.e. intense, sudden, uncontrollable, unexpected experiences that have an extremely negative impact (Brewin et al., 2000; Carlson, 1997; Carlson & Dalenberg, 2000; Foa et al., 1992; Ogawa et al., 1997). Interpersonal violence events, which cause physical wounds or represent a threat for the individual's safety, entail a higher risk of traumatisation compared to other highly stressful experiences, such as, for instance, natural disasters (APA, 1994; Breslau et al., 1999; Darves-Bornoz et al., 1998; Holbrook et al., 2002). Those events that are not life-threatening but fall within the sphere of attachment relationships – i.e. the loss of a loved one (Waelde et al., 2001), deception or betrayal by a parenting figure (Freyd, 1996) – increase the risk of traumatisation. Child abuse often includes all these factors.

During childhood, interpersonal violence is often accompanied by neglect (Draijer, 1990; Nijenhuis et al., 2003). Even though it is also present in adult relationships, neglect represents a form of traumatisation where the required physical caretaking or an appropriate emotional support – like soothing when crying or the reparation of meaningful affect relationships – is missing. These are fundamental requisites for child development; however, there are situations in adulthood when they are relevant any way, such as, for example, immediately after a potentially traumatising event (van der Hart et al., 2006).

A prolonged and consistent exposure to stressful factors such as child abuse seems to exert the most harmful effects on the victims. Chronic traumatisation highly exposes to post-traumatic syndromes and to more serious and pervasive symptoms, among them substance abuse (Dube et al., 2001) and suicide attempts (Dube et al., 2003). These symptoms do not only relate to the psychic functioning. In fact, they can also appear at neurophysiological levels considering that brain development and neuro-endocrine functions are seriously compromised (Anda et al., 2006; Dube et al., 2003; Breslau et al., 1995; Draijer & Boon, 1999; Glaser, 2000; Hillis et al., 2004; Nijenhuis et al., 2003; Ozer et al., 2003; Perry, 1994; Schore, 2003). Chronic traumatisation is one of the factors that determine the development of more complex forms of structural dissociation. The lack of social support accounts for a considerable risk variable in the development of some post-traumatic syndromes (Brewin et al., 2000; Ozer et al., 2003). This happens in children even more, given that they totally depend on the adult's help in their integration of difficult experiences. Soothing, support and caretaking are essential to maintain and enhance the individual's psychic efficiency (Runtz, 1997), partly thanks to their soothing effect (Schore, 1994, 2003) and to their beneficial effect on the immune system (Uchino *et al.*, 1996).

The diagnosis of post-traumatic stress disorder (PTSD) and acute stress disorder (ASD) are the only diagnoses to consider the aetiological aspect among their diagnostic criteria, hence, trauma (APA, 2000). However, they are not enough for a specific list of symptoms that are often detected in clients suffering from various disorders and all with developmental stories characterised by relational traumas. Several clinicians and researchers, experts in trauma-related pathologies, have proposed different, similar diagnoses that would allow identifying in adults those psychopathological outcome of repeated relational and cumulative traumas experienced in childhood: developmental traumatic disorder (van der Kolk, 2005) and complex post-traumatic stress disorder (Herman, 1992), to mention a few. Actually, experts seem to agree on the fact that the vulnerability following such developmental experiences mainly concerns the integration functions of memory and awareness, and thus, it causes some dissociative symptoms as shown by Liotti and Farina in their book *Sviluppi traumatici* (Liotti and Farina, 2011). Some meta-analyses have isolated a few relevant factors that can predict PTSD in adults. They include previous traumatisation (accumulated in time), particularly chronic forms of child abuse, previous psychological adaptation, existing psychopathology in the family history, perception of life threats during the traumatic events, peri-traumatic emotional reactions, peri-traumatic dissociation and lacking social support (Brewin *et al.*, 2000; Emily *et al.*, 2003; Holbrook *et al.*, 2002; Ozer *et al.*, 2003). Abused children often show a combination of all these factors (van der Hart *et al.*, 2006). The onset of disorders following a trauma depends on the victim's age upon traumatisation. The younger the victim, the higher the possibilities to develop a post-traumatic syndrome. This happens for PTDS, complex PTSD, borderline personality disorder following a trauma, not otherwise specified dissociative disorders (DDNOS), sub-type I (Boon and Draijer, 1993; Brewin *et al.*, 2000; Herman *et al.*, 1989; Liotti and Farina, 2000; Nijenhuis *et al.*, 1998; Ogawa *et al.*, 1997; Roth *et al.*, 1997).

Chronic traumatisation starting in infancy follows different paths compared to other types of traumatisation, both because the child's mental efficiency and psychobiological development have not reached maturity yet and because the child still needs care and support (van der Hart *et al.*, 2006).

4.3   Interpersonal trauma in children

Children's exposure to interpersonal traumatic stress factors is extremely frequent. In fact, this phenomenon has been labelled as a silent epidemic. All over the world, approximately one child out of three is estimated to be a victim of physical abuses; about one girl out of four and one boy out of five is a victim of sexual abuses (Anda *et al.*, 1999; Felitti *et al.*, 1998; Putnam, 2003; United Nations, 2006). Many researches have proven that exposure to interpersonal trauma can chronically alter the individual's biological, cognitive, psychological and social development in a pervasive way (Burns *et al.*, 1998; Cook *et al.*, 2005; Spinazzola *et al.*, 2005). Children can experience many forms of relational traumatic experiences in addition to physical and sexual abuses. Unfortunately, child abuse can occur in several forms, among them aggression, kidnapping, bullying and neglect.

Even though we can use the term *victimisation* to define the victims of natural disasters, serious medical diseases or accidents, the reference is most frequently made to people who are victims of interpersonal trauma. In the cases of interpersonal victimisation, hostility, trust betrayal, the feeling of the experienced injustice and the immorality of abusive behaviours seem to account for the most significant factors compared to what happens to the victims of accidents, the people suffering from organic diseases or involved in natural disasters (Finkelhor, 2008). No psychiatric diagnostic label can currently describe the complex pool of symptoms at best, which research has proven to be typical in children who have experienced interpersonal trauma. When experiencing trauma, children may feel that their sense of safety and the foreseeability of present and future are undermined. The realisation of their own needs and the attainment of the main developmental steps may be compromised, with the following damage to the elements making up the psychological functioning: the sense of self-effectiveness, self-esteem, the ability to regulate emotions, the world of interpersonal relationships (Verardo, 2016). The stress possibly following the traumatic experience often leads to the development of typical disorders, such as PTSD.

PTSD may not be able to include all symptoms originating from a trauma satisfactorily, and this is true in children in particular. Some research suggests that PTSD is the fifth (Ackerman *et al.*, 1998) or tenth (Copeland *et al.*, 2007) child disorder, which shows up following a traumatic experience. Co-morbid diagnosis is then quite frequent, and it is no exception: 40% of children with a trauma history report at least one additional diagnosis, as mood disorder, anxiety disorder or disruptive behaviour disorder. This relationship between symptoms and diagnosis is exacerbated even more when the child is exposed to a high number or to different types of traumatic stressors (Copeland *et al.*, 2007). Consistently with these research outcomes, some epidemiological and clinical studies have shown that the number and complexity of symptoms and diagnoses during development grow when the number and type of traumatic events they are exposed to increase (D'Andrea *et al.*, 2015). Even if other factors – i.e. chronicity, the violation of physical and emotional boundaries, the betrayal of trust by the perpetrator – are among the elements connected to victimisation and they strongly affect the risk and severity of post-traumatic symptoms and the functional impairment in children and adolescents, it was proven that the simple exposure to a higher number of victimisation types may affect the development of complex, severe symptoms within a wide scope of psychiatric disorders (Finkelhor *et al.*, 2009).

Studies on the consequences of child abuse and cumulative trauma as relational traumatic experience have shown that children and adolescents can develop severe chronical difficulties in regulating affects and behaviours, in attention and cognitive processes, in interpersonal relations and in the meaning attributions to their own and third-party emotions. In addition, it was suggested that early traumatic experiences could lead to dissociative states and symptoms in adulthood (D'Andrea *et al.*, 2015). Talking about *interpersonal trauma*, reference can be made to the different forms of maltreatment, interpersonal violence, abuse, attacks and neglect experienced by the child and the adolescent, which occur within the family. They include physical, sexual and emotional abuses, incest, different forms of serious neglect (physical, medical and emotional neglect), experience of witnessed domestic violence and the incidence of serious, pervasive breaches in the caregiving behaviours originated by the parents' mental diseases, substance abuse, involvement in criminal activities, sudden separation and traumatic loss. In addition, these terms will be used to refer to the aggressions perpetrated by peers at school, to harassment and serious bullying.

This complex definition of interpersonal trauma originates from the description used by the National Child Traumatic Stress Network (NCTSN), developed thanks to some longitudinal research conducted on a large sample of children with a trauma history (Pynoos *et al.*, 2008). This is similar to the categorisation given by the National Child Abuse and Neglect Data System (NCANDS: U.S. Department of Health and Human Services, 2011).

4.4   Adverse childhood experiences (ACE)

Many observations have been made on the repercussions that adverse childhood experiences can have on psychic health; however, in fact, these experiences affect physical health as well (Verardo, 2016).

This was shown by an important study lasting 16 years, which involved 17,000 people in the USA, conducted by the Department of Preventive Medicine at Kaiser Permanent in San Diego. The study proved the correlation between the exposure to (emotional, physical or sexual) abuse during infancy, dysfunctional family situations or physical or emotional neglect and the development of diseases during adulthood (i.e. cancer, COPD, liver diseases, CHD, diabetes, chronic headache, depression) and risky behaviours (i.e. substance abuse and suicide) (Felitti *et al.*, 1998). Such correlation was demonstrated by administering the ACE (adverse childhood experience) questionnaire, which includes questions on different forms of abuse, such as the presence of mental diseases inside the family, a relative's substance addiction and criminal and violent behaviours against the mother by one of the family members. Questions were added on the child's conditions and feelings of neglect and rejection by his/her attachment figures.

All these experiences had the same impact on vulnerability to diseases, and an ACE score was adopted to express the number of negative experiences up to 18 years of age. The higher the score, the more diseases were reported. How can we explain this phenomenon? Long periods of stress stimulate our orthosympathetic system and increase the cortisol level in the blood, thus inhibiting the immune system and making us more vulnerable to diseases. In addition, cortisol increases those substances that foster inflammation and that are responsible for alterations in the circulatory system.

The attachment theory and the research on abuse provide some clues on how the abuse cycle can be broken and on how it is possible to benefit from the presence of new support connections even when there have been several and repeated negative experiences during childhood. Among adults with one or more adverse experiences, those who reported having three or more effective family figures or friends they could talk to about their own problems and who could support them showed a lower vulnerability to depressive states and they were in a better health state (Verardo, 2016).

4.5 Abuse and sexual harassment

Literature reports that sexual abuse in childhood could represent a major pathogenic factor. The reaction to abuse may vary a lot from child to child. According to many authors, this depends on several factors, such as the child's cognitive ability, the duration and frequency of the abuse, the type of coercion, the relationship between the child and the perpetrator, the type of abuse and the family members' response to the child (Koch, 1980; Walker *et al.*, 1988, Wodarski and Jhonson, 1988). It was assumed that both psychological and social characteristics represent some resources for the victims: self-confidence, a good knowledge of how sex works, the possibility to count on the support by meaningful adult figures, a strong basic personality, some success areas in life, some clear and concrete goals to attain (Finkelhor and Baron, 1986). According to Finkelhor's theory, child sexual abuse includes traumatic sexualisation and impotence, and it originates fear associated with anxiety symptoms, i.e. nightmares, sleep disturbance, psychosomatic symptoms and dissociative reactions, which, in some cases, may even meet the PTSD criteria (De Leo & Kilmartin, 1999). According to Green (1994), children who are victims of sexual abuses can have two different adaptation styles: one seeking control through the active reiteration of the experienced trauma, while another only addressing it by avoiding sexual stimuli.

4.6 Short-term consequences

Children do not usually have specific knowledge of sex and sexual intercourse; hence, they cannot give their consent to a sexual intercourse with an adult. Many children experience sexual abuse for years; however, while they are growing up, they become more aware of the fact that something is wrong, and they can suddenly understand what is happening (Petruccelli and Scardaccione, 1998).

The adaptation problems the victim must face can be summarised in two moments: an acute, short-term phase of total disorganisation, whose main symptom is fear; and a second, chronical, long-term phase two or three weeks after the attack, when the victim re-organises their own lifestyle (Burgess and Holmstrom, 1974). Pre-school children cannot understand their experience; thus, they cannot communicate what has happened verbally. In fact, they do not master the vocabulary related to adult sexual behaviour. This leaves them in a state of confusion and disorientation regarding the abuse experience (Urquiza and Capra, 1990).

Particularly, the symptoms in a child who was sexually abused in pre-school age include physical and behavioural symptoms. Physical symptoms include physical disorders, sleep disorders, nightmares, enuresis, eating disorders and headache (Browne and Finkelhor, 1986; Rimsza et al., 1988; Dent, 1993; Fullerton et al., 1995; Krakow et al., 1995; Sexual Assault Crisis Center, 1998). Do not forget psychic consequences due to somatic disorders too (Friedrich and Schaefer, 1995).

The most evident short-term psycho-behavioural symptoms are as follows: anxiety, extreme shyness, fear to fail, retiring attitude, silence, non-communicative behaviour, hostility and aggression with peers, low self-esteem, learning difficulties, intense rage, phobias, age-inappropriate social behaviours, escape from home, fear to meet specific people and to visit specific places, school and disciplinary issues, regressive behaviours, infantilism, oppositional-contrasting behaviours, problematic relationship with peers, depression, isolation, delinquency, substance abuse, suicide attempts, early marriage (Browne and Finkelhor, 1986; Duenas, 1986; Rimsza et al., 1988; Vargo and Jacobs, 1988; Hanks et al., 1988; Lynch, 1988; Hall and Hall, 1989; Urquiza and Capra, 1990; Dent, 1993; Fenwick, 1994; Fullerton et al., 1995; Krakow et al., 1995; Sexual Assault Crisis Center, 1998).

In addition, clinical literature describes some cases in which the victims tend to have self-endangering behaviours, such as self-mutilation, suicidal ideations or attempts and sundry self-destructive behaviours (Browne and Finkelhor, 1986; Rimsza et al., 1988; Urquiza and Capra, 1990; Fullerton et al., 1995; Sexual Assault Crisis Center, 1998). It was also observed that children who have been sexually abused report a sudden worsening in their school performance, disturbed cognitive processes, anxiety, growing depression and post-traumatic stress disorder, little confidence and phobia towards adults, sexual pseudo-maturity and inappropriate sexual behaviours (Browne and Finkelhor, 1986; Bastianon and De Benedetti Gaddini, 1987; Hanks et al., 1988; Lynch, 1988; Rimsza et al., 1988; Urquiza and Capra, 1990; Finkelhor, 1990; Cosentino et al., 1995; Mayall and Gold, 1995; Oberlander, 1995; Fullerton et al., 1995; Brand et al., 1996).

As concerns the negative impacts on sexual behaviour, some authors believe that experiencing sexual abuse can cause a disinhibition effect on the child's sexual behaviour. Thus, the following are frequent: manifest and excessive masturbation, exhibition of their own genitals, attempt to introduce objects into their genitals and sexual aggression, highly sexualised behaviours and plays (Cosentino et al., 1995; Mayall and Gold, 1995; Petruccelli and Scardaccione, 1998). The child victims of sexual abuse tend to sexualise all their relationships since they have associated sexuality to the attentions other people can have towards them. They use sexual behaviours to manipulate others, and they often find it difficult to give and receive love as adults (De Leo & Kilmartin, 1999). In addition, they can find it difficult to show their anger due to experienced irritation towards the adults that did not protect them and towards the abuse perpetrator.

We have observed that children show signs of depression and tend to 'sacrifice' themselves personally, either through a passive withdrawal or through violently self-destructive behaviours (De Leo & Kilmartin, 1999). The consequences on the sexual behaviour of abused children include sexual disorders, inappropriate sexual behaviour, hypersexuality, sexual acting out and gender confusion. In particular, reference here is to male victims of sexual abuse by male adults, who often show confusion concerning their sexual identity and their sexual preferences (De Leo & Kilmartin, 1999). A strategy used by the victim to address trauma is to identify with the perpetrator: by re-acting the sexual behaviour he has suffered, the victim becomes active and no more passive, thus trying to control the anxiety and anguish caused by the abuse trauma. Some children can swing between identification with the victim's role and identification with the perpetrator's role (Urquiza and Capra, 1990; Cosentino et al., 1995; Petruccelli and Scardaccione, 1998).

Sexually abused children more often show a poor self-image, growing feelings of guilt, shame, sense of being different from the others, no self-confidence, self-perception as a victim, reduced self-esteem, depression, somatic disorders, social withdrawal, immaturity and obsessive-compulsive behaviours. Emotional stress is a common reaction to sexual victimisation both in males and in females (Urquiza and Capra, 1990; Sexual Assault Crisis Center, 1998).

4.7 Long-term consequences

Many studies conducted in the last decades have confirmed the connection between childhood sexual abuses and the later presence of a wide range of symptoms.

Long-term effects following the acute phase of reaction differ from child to child as per the symptoms. Consequences, in fact, depend on a number of factors, i.e. age, cognitive ability, the child's psychological characteristics, the family's reaction to the harassment and the very same nature of the abuse (Koch, 1980; De Young, 1982; Walker et al., 1988; Wodarski and Jhonson, 1988; Cross et al., 1994). The most negative effects that provoke serious disorders in adult life depend on the type of experienced abuse, its frequency and duration (Cross et al., 1994).

The consequences of a sexual abuse in childhood must be associated with the victim's age. Younger children somatise trauma with different psychosomatic symptoms, which can persist for some time after the abuse. When the abuse is perpetrated between 9 and 10 years of age, the victims are aware of the abuse reality they are experiencing, they feel shame and they can be induced to silence more easily. During adolescence, the victims can escape and enact sexual promiscuity and suicide attempts (De Leo & Kilmartin, 1999). The most typical long-term consequences include sleep disorders, which can show up in many forms: the victim can find it difficult to go to bed or fall asleep. Quite often, enuresis and encopresis appear, and there can be nightmares and sleepwalking in adulthood. The symptoms in adult victims of child abuses are described as characterised by sleep and eating disorders, irritability and aggression, chronical anger, agoraphobia, depression, sense of isolation, feeling guilty for the experienced abuse, unhealthy attachment to meaningful figures, self-destructive behaviours, suicide attempts, low self-esteem and interpersonal problems characterised by unstable relationships (Browne and Finkelhor, 1986; Briere et al., 1988; Kiser et al., 1988; Fromuth and Burkhart, 1989;

Olson, 1990; Terr, 1991; Bagley *et al.*, 1994; Lisak, 1994; Simpson, 1994; Wolfe *et al.*, 1994; Collings, 1995; Peters and Range, 1995; Brand *et al.*, 1996; Lisak, 1997).

Green observed that all clients who have experienced sexual abuses in their childhood reported exaggerated anxiety in adulthood, which was enacted through hypervigilance, failed control over their own urges, inappropriate social behaviours and depressive symptoms, including sense of solitude and no self-confidence. According to this author, the victims survive trauma by reiterating the abuse in dreams, fantasies, aggressive plays, self-destructive behaviours and delinquency. As regards the effect on adult sexuality, we must first analyse the differences from gender to gender. Considering the female population, clinical studies have shown significantly higher dysfunctional sexual behaviours in abused women compared to the control groups (De Leo & Kilmartin, 1999). The sexual problems presented by abused women can include the following: difficulty to have a climax, inhibited desire and sexual arousal, sex-aversive feelings and fear of intimacy, sexual frigidity and inability to establish long-lasting affect and sexual relationships, tendency to sexual promiscuity and prostitution, a compulsive sexual desire (Herman, 1981; Browne and Finkelhor, 1986; Fromuth, 1986; Alexander and Lupfer, 1987; Bastianon and De Benedetti Gaddini, 1987; Canepa, 1987; Jehu, 1988; Greenwald *et al.*, 1990; Urquiza and Capra, 1990; Belkin *et al.*, 1994; Bray, 1994; Simpson *et al.*, 1994; Miller *et al.*, 1995; O'Hagan, 1995; Oberlander, 1995; Brand *et al.*, 1996; Mullen *et al.*, 1996).

Collings (1995) compared a group of abused males with a control group and found that an experience of abuse implying physical contact leads to more severe effects on the psychological and sexual functioning compared to other forms of abuse with no physical contact. In fact, Myers (1989) states that abused men are more likely to report erection difficulties, primary and secondary delayed ejaculation and fragile and unstable sexual identity, thus often developing a real homophobia and presenting a distorted, negative body image coupled with a low self-esteem and no self-confidence. Some authors suggest that the victim's inappropriate sexual behaviour can represent a process by which the sexual activity becomes – under pathological conditions – a way to express their own main affect needs. Pursuant to this approach, a dysfunctional sexualised behaviour would be the outcome of a social learning (De Leo & Petruccelli, 1999).

The adults who have suffered sexual abuses in childhood show disrespect towards themselves and feelings of contamination, worthlessness and corruption. When the abuse was perpetrated, they felt abandoned. Thus, they are in search of continuous attentions and care, and consequently, they recreate essentially abusing relationships. This is the reason why adults who were sexually abused as children often perpetrate physical and sexual abuse against their own children. The physical affection these parents feel for their children is not aimed at taking care of them. It has a sexual meaning. In some cases, mothers unconsciously enact seduction attitudes to maintain their children's discipline (Petruccelli and Scardaccione, 1998; De Leo & Kilmartin, 1999). Although women in general tend more towards depression and suicide attempts, not only abused women enact self-endangering behaviours. Men also express their discomfort in a similar way, particularly through anxiety, depression and low self-esteem (De Leo & Laan, 1999). In many cases, the abuse of toxic substances, particularly alcohol and drugs, starts shortly after the violence, and this allows the victim to escape both present and past situations (Simpson *et al.*, 1994; Petruccelli and Scardaccione, 1998). Women tend to develop borderline personality traits more compared to men (impulsivity, failure in their social role, intolerance to frustration, depressive states). Men mostly develop antisocial personality disorders (De Leo & Laan, 1999).

Chapter 5

EMDR therapy

Elena Isola and Bruna Maccarrone

5.1 Introduction

One of the most important novelties of the last 20 years in the field of psycho-traumatology and psychotherapy has been the wide dissemination of EMDR (Eye Movement Desensitisation and Reprocessing). EMDR is a psychotherapeutic method now widely spread and applied in Italy and in the world. Founded on the AIP (adaptive information processing) model, EMDR postulates the existence of an innate system to process information that would lead to good functioning, adaptation and meaning building, which can somehow make life and relationships with other people possible. EMDR allows access to those frozen, partially processed memories stored in a dysfunctional way in the neural networks, thus allowing their unlocking and reprocessing, the completion of their processing and their reconsolidation in an adaptive and functional way. According to AIP, maladaptively stored memories lie at the basis of the onset of psychological disorders.

Currently, the easiest explanation to describe the observable clinical effects consists in considering EMDR as a method used fundamentally to access the memories of traumatic experiences, process them and lead them to an adaptive resolution. Such memories lie at the basis of the client's psychological disorders in the form of information stored in a non-functional way inside the memory (Balbo, 2015). The processing of these memories and their integration into wider adaptive networks allows their transformation and reconsolidation. An adaptive resolution takes place when connections are built during processing with appropriate associations and the client uses the experience in a constructive way; thus, it is integrated into a positive emotional and cognitive scheme (Shapiro, 1995).

EMDR was created as an innovative technique that utilizes eye movements stimulated bilaterally in an alternated way to facilitate and accelerate the desensitisation and processing of disturbing traumatic events (Shapiro, 1995; Fernandez *et al.*, 2011). EMDR has now turned into a refined, complex psychotherapeutic method and approach targeted to treat most psychopathological disorders, even severe ones. Human beings have an innate capacity to heal from both emotional and physical wounds. In fact, there seems to exist a neurological balance that allows information processing to head towards an adaptive resolution. However, some highly traumatic

DOI: 10.4324/9781003508670-6

experiences can destabilise this system. EMDR focuses on the memory of the traumatic experiences, which contributed to develop the pathology, or the discomfort shown by the client. The processing of the traumatic experience is activated by the alternated bilateral stimulation that the therapist performs while the client focuses on the components that make up the memory of the traumatic experience.

In the last years, the effects of this form of short treatment have also allowed neurobiologists to have a 'look inside the brain'. To this purpose, over a dozen researches were conducted supported by brain imaging (i.e. MRI – magnetic resonance imaging techniques) to document how the EMDR treatment changes it concretely. For example, it was established that the brain structure in charge of controlling memory (the hippocampus) shrinks in the people who suffer from post-traumatic stress disorder. For some time, it was believed that such shrinkage – being an organic change – would be a permanent pathological condition. Magnetic resonance examinations have shown, instead, that the hippocampus growth is possible again. However, even if the effectiveness of EMDR has been widely demonstrated, the reason for its working is still open to debate, just like all other forms of psychotherapy. Since this is a complex process, many factors are implied, and thus, the number of related research projects is increasing. In fact, the use of eye movements in therapy has stirred the interest of many researchers (Dworkin, 2010; Shapiro and Laliotis, 2011) who have explored the changes occurring with eye movements only. They have shown that in the people who keep in mind some disturbing memories or fears about their future, the series of eye movements originates a reduction in the emotional suffering and in the vividness of the disturbing images, thus producing changes in the thoughts and a higher memory precision too.

Of course, the effectiveness of EMDR therapy and the duration of the occurring changes is not based only on eye movements or on other forms of bilateral stimulation but on a more articulated procedure, which represents an intervention protocol: eye movements are clearly a fundamental integrative part of it.

During therapy sessions, clients are awake, and they keep full control of their own capacities. The work is performed during the treatment sessions, with no need to do homework. EMDR consists in a dual attention task, during which the client is invited to focus internally on the different parts of a disturbing memory (the worst image, the negative cognition, the emotion and the physical sensation) according to a standard protocol, which is now widely consolidated and proved. At the same time, the client is asked to follow an external stimulus, the therapist's fingers moving from right to left, or to receive alternative tactile stimulation (tapping). The therapist accesses the disturbing memory, restarts the information processing system, follows the process and monitors its effects without interfering on the contents and direction of the processing path followed by the client. During a session, new connections are created in a rapid and spontaneous way with the neural networks containing the adaptive material, i.e. new insights, more positive memories, pleasant emotions and feelings that help the client feel the traumatic memory in a different perspective and consider the event and their own self in a very different way compared to the beginning.

5.2   EMDR as an evidence-based therapy

Numerous research projects conducted in the past 20 years have led to label EMDR as an evidence-based treatment, which is effective to treat trauma as in many clinical guidelines issued by national professional and mental health care organisations. EMDR has been awarded many important international awards, and therapists from different clinical approaches use it.

In 2000, EMDR was added to the guidelines of the International Society for Traumatic Stress Studies as the therapy with the most numerous scientific evidences. In 2001, the United Kingdom Department of Health also added it to evidence-based therapies in the guidelines for clinical practice. In 2002, the Israeli National Council for Mental Health acknowledged EMDR as one of the three most recommended methods for the treatment of the victims of terror attacks. In 2004, the US Veterans Health Affair National Clinical Practice Guideline Council and the Ministry of Defence included it in their guidelines for the treatment of PTSD, and in the same year, the Guidelines for Clinical Practice by the American Psychiatric Association acknowledged its efficacy too. In 2005, NICE (the National Institute for Clinical Excellence) likewise defined cognitive-behavioural therapy (CBT) and EMDR as the two best methods to treat PTSD in adults because they are both empirically founded and, hence, evidence-based. In 2007, the *British Journal of Psychiatry* reported EMDR, with trauma-focused cognitive-behavioural therapy, as a preferred approach in the field of trauma. In 2013, the World Health Organisation (WHO, 2013) stated that cognitive-behavioural therapy and EMDR were the two therapies recommended for children, adolescents and adults suffering from PTSD and other specifically stress-related conditions.

The Centre for Mental Health of the US Government Department of Health listed EMDR among the treatments suggested not only for PTSD but also for other anxiety disorders, for depression and for the promotion of mental health. This acknowledgment was based on the quality of research and scientific publications that prove the effectiveness of EMDR and the absence of any damaging, secondary or undesired effects after its application.

Some important meta-analyses (Bisson and Andrew, 2007) show that EMDR produces therapeutic effects equivalent to those of other methods that are more often investigated in scientific projects, like cognitive-behavioural therapy (Faretta, 2014). Many studies show the effectiveness of EMDR with a wide range of disorders, including phobias (De Jongh et al., 1999; De Jongh et al., 2002), panic disorders (Goldstein et al., 2000; Fernandez and Faretta, 2007), general anxiety disorders (Gauvreau and Bouchard, 2008), conduct and self-esteem disorders (Soberman et al., 2002; Solomon and Rando, 2007), body dysmorphic disorder (Brown et al., 1997), olfactory reference syndrome (McGoldrick et al., 2008), sexual dysfunctions (Wernik, 1993), paedophilia (Ricci et al., 2006), performance anxiety (Barker and Barker, 2007), chronic pain (Grant and Threlfo, 2002), headaches (Marcus, 2008) and hallucinations (Schneider et al., 2008; Tinker and Wilson, 2006; de Roos et al., 2010). Some neurobiological studies have shown changes before and after

EMDR, together with a remission of trauma symptoms (Lamprecht *et al.*, 2004; Lansing *et al.*, 2005; Levin *et al.*, 1999). The assessments made during EMDR studies have demonstrated that the level of compliance with the treatment procedures and protocols is positively associated with the level of effects exerted by the same treatment (Maxfield and Hyer, 2002; Shapiro, 1999).

Pagani and his team (Pagani *et al.*, 2011, 2012) have used EEG to investigate the functional reaction of some clients with PTSD before, during and after treatment with EMDR. By comparing the EEG of clients during the first and the last EMDR session, they highlighted a higher activation in the temporo-occipital cortex, mainly on the left side, during the latter. The prevalent limbic activation during the typical EMDR alternated bilateral stimulation, which is present in the orbito-frontal cortex (OFC), in the prefrontal cortex (PFC) and in the anterior cingulate cortex (ACC) during the first EMDR session in the acute phase, later moves to the temporo-occipital regions after treatment. Traumatic memories thus move from an implicit sub-cortical to an explicit cortical state, where different brain regions contribute to processing and reprocessing the experience. A normalisation of the activation after trauma processing was highlighted, which can be interpreted as the neurobiological related effect of the improving symptoms (Faretta, 2014).

In addition to reducing the most evident emotional disturbances and symptoms, during EMDR sessions, clients experience a great variety of reactions. They show the emergence of a large reorganisation that translates into a change in the affect regulation and in the personality characteristics (Brown and Shapiro, 2006; Korn and Leeds, 2002; Zabukovec and Huber, 1995) and into changes in the cognitive organisation, which shows up in the number of positive memories that can be evoked after treatment (Sprang, 2001).

5.3   How does EMDR work? The general characteristics of the system

Several assumptions have been made on how EMDR works and many studies have investigated its possible mechanisms to now: eye movements have proven their ability to regulate and reduce physiological hyper-arousal by probably rebalancing the sympathetic and parasympathetic unbalance generated by traumatic events. EMDR increases the parasympathetic activity and slows down both the heart and the breathing rate. In addition, it fosters the integration between implicit and explicit memory, between semantic and episodic memory, thus enhancing autobiographical memory.

Moreover, data is now available to show an increase in the narrative consistency in the reconstruction of their own attachment history (Zaccagnino *et al.*, 2015) obtained with EMDR.

More and more studies have recently been conducted to show that EMDR leads to a normalisation of the activity of slow brain waves in the two cortical hemispheres and thus to a new synchronisation of the two hemispheres (Winson, 1993; Pagani *et al.*, 2012; Farina *et al.*, 2014). EMDR would lead to a normalisation of cortisol levels in the blood, too, which are known to be altered in post-traumatic syndromes (Levine and Landon, 2002). These studies allow us to assume that EMDR is closely related to the world of scientific research and to psychophysiology studies.

5.3.1   Big 'T' traumas and small 't' traumas

The psychological trauma can be considered as a 'wound in the soul', i.e. an experience with such an intense, negative emotional impact to demand special care to heal (Fernandez et al., 2011). Not all traumas are the same, and they do not bring about the same consequences. In fact, we can identify two main types of traumatic events: big 'T' traumas and small 't' traumas.

Big 'T' traumas are the result of a single, well-recognisable and well-defined event in time, for instance, natural disasters (like earthquakes, floods and tsunamis), potentially lethal accidents, attacks, the diagnosis of life-endangering diseases, miscarriages and rapes, which have threatened the individual's life or the life of the loved ones. The reaction to these events should have caused *fear*, *horror* and *sense of vulnerability* in the person, according to the definition of trauma provided in the Diagnostic and Statistical Manual of Mental Disorders, *DSM-5* (2014), where PTSD (post-traumatic stress disorder) is described.

On the opposite, small 't' psychological traumas are the outcome of a series of disturbing events, each of which does not generate the perception of a threat to the person's life per se. Even though such experiences may seem little relevant if compared to more serious and catastrophic events, they can affect the normal development of personality when they reiterate during one's life. In addition, they can negatively affect the individual's concept of self and the expectations on how the world works. Examples include the experience of humiliations, denigrations and devaluations by parents and teachers.

5.3.2   The body in EMDR

In EMDR, the body plays a major role since it 'talks in a clearer way compared to words' (Gonzalez Vazquez and Mosquera, 2012). EMDR helps the client come into contact with their own body and with those feelings, which sometimes represent the only memory trace of a dissociated traumatic experience that cannot be accessed as a biographical and explicit memory. EMDR allows processing, and integrating these fragments inside a more organised and complete memory in which the experience – even though a negative one – does not generate discomfort anymore and takes up more adaptive meanings for oneself and the world, thus paving the way to new experiences and restarting the flow of their own existence.

The main goal is to foster the integration of the neural networks containing the maladaptive materials with more adaptive information so that the client can reach a more consistent sense of self (Gomez, 2013). Before tackling and treating the traumatic experience with EMDR, clients are assessed carefully and accurately to check if they are ready to start work on the trauma, which is preceded by a preparation phase. To this purpose, specific techniques and procedures are used to stabilise the client so that they can tolerate the impact with the emotions connected to the traumatic memory without feeling overwhelmed so they can perceive the safety and containment of the therapeutic setting. During the last phase in the protocol, the 'body is given the last word' because it is the final source of information showing if the processing has taken place and the negative traces of the traumatic memories have disappeared.

5.3.3   The treatment of trauma-based sexual dysfunctions

Sexual dysfunctions can be read as the best adaptive response an individual has found in a precise moment in life to solve a specific problem. Unresolved existential situations, traumas, relational issues, prohibitions and orders inherited from their own family and personal experience are at the basis of several forms of discomfort and suffering. This is even stronger when they relate to such intimate and meaningful aspects of a person's life, such as affect and sexuality. Sexuality is a relational place where much comes into play: trust, contact, relation to the body, being worthy, being able to let go and to be able to receive and give what you feel you need.

Sexual disorders of a psychological nature are characterised by internal dynamics, personal or relational experiences that interfere negatively with the possibility that a meeting can come up to a positive and gratifying way. Among them, the presence of 'internal prohibitions' and sense of guilt, which prevent the person from accepting pleasure, the difficulty to relax and to experience body sensations, the fear to trust other people, the fear for refusal and for failure (performance anxiety), individual problems connected to anxiety, stress, nervousness, mood disorders that prevent the normal physical and psychic dynamics of a sexual contact to happen, beliefs and false myths that prevent a satisfactory contact, fixations and fixed, dysfunctional cognitive schemes. Many experts believe that the origin of sexual dysfunctions lies in a meaningful correlation when clients have been sexually traumatised by an event in early infancy, when they were not emotionally equipped to react to it correctly, and when the first attempt to come in contact with the other sex – a very critical moment – was a failure or an experience generating fears or humiliations. The destructive potential of a serious trauma like being a victim of abuse or incestuous seductions in childhood is evident.

However, the first failures of a young adult, even though not that dramatic, often start an escalation of anxiety, further failures and desperation, which can prejudice a person's sexual functioning throughout their lifetime. Such sexual failures can provoke very intense emotional reactions that the young adult loses his ability to judge and logically assess the reasons for his failures or *defaillance*. Many clients cannot see their problem as a temporary, understandable reaction to stress, which originates from the fact that they have been upset or too little informed on the dynamics of sexuality, so they may feel discouraged and scared up to desperation.

Pain and frustration for an initial failure can affect the individual who is then prone to experiment anticipatory anxiety, which will later lead to new failures. Alternatively, the individual may escape anxiety by avoiding having any other sexual encounter, for some time, at least. Once again, reluctance to sex is strengthened by reduced anxiety and persists even if its effects are negative, considering that, when a person renounces to sex, he is deprived of the occasion to have other positive corrective experiences later. Thus, he is deprived of the possibility to eliminate anxiety. Initial sexual failures do not often translate into a permanent sexual inappropriateness if the person does not avoid other sexual occasions later on.

If we analyse the source of the problem correctly as a temporary reaction due to stress and no experience, if the person regains self-confidence, the effects of the early failure will be rapidly cancelled by positive sexual episodes that will extinguish the anticipatory anxiety originated by the negative consequences of the first critical attempts. Unfortunately, these strengthening and neutralisation factors are not always available. The combination of different clinical interventions can allow responding appropriately to those disorders, which imply aspects that are more dysfunctional, and in all those situations that require a multidimensional intervention. Particularly, when a traumatic experience has originated a sexual disorder, traditional psychotherapy may be coupled with EMDR. In this way, it is possible to intervene on those experiences, which the body keeps in memory and that keep on exercising a pervasive influence on the presence even though they are referred to the past.

No doubt, sexuality refers to the emotional as well as physical intimate sphere. Hence, somatic and emotional implications as well are strongly relevant in the clinical assessment and treatment of sexual disorders.

5.4   Case conceptualisation in EMDR

As observed here earlier, the EMDR treatment is based on the AIP criteria according to which the cause of a dysfunction (emotions, feelings, behaviours and beliefs) depends on the memories of unprocessed aetiological events. Thus, after carefully defining current dysfunctional behaviours, emotions and negative beliefs in addition to any other specific symptoms, we investigate each single symptom with the client and ask, 'When was the first disturbing moment that originated the dysfunction? Whom did you learn it from? Where did you learn it?' And so on. 'What was the international, social and family situation like at the time of the first event? When was the first time you remember you felt this way?' (Shapiro, 2001, page 106). The EMDR literature recommends the 'emotional scan' (Shapiro, 1995) to identify the relevant target memories for the EMDR treatment. Alternatively, a procedural variant can be used name the 'float-back technique' (Browning, 1999). This procedure can be used when the client cannot easily identify an early target memory for processing (Shapiro, 2001, page 433), and it is based on the 'bridge emotion' or somatic bridge principles. It is a form of free associations that start from the client's current emotional experiences and in which the client receives specific general instructions. The basic assumption is that the client's neural network will show – based on emotional affinities – what target memory or pivot event is relevant. The client is asked to recall a situation during which the symptoms or problems have often shown up and to identify a corresponding image, a negative cognition and an emotion. Then the client is asked to go back in time and find a relevant past event when he felt or thought the same way.

The float-back technique always uses the following gradual procedure:

- 'When was the last time you felt this way?'
- 'Focus on the image that comes to your mind and on the thoughts that come up with this image'.
- 'Where can you feel it in your body?'
- 'Focus your attention on the image and on the emotions and allow your mind to bring you back to the first time when you felt this way'.

5.5 The eight phases in the EMDR treatment

Phase 1: History taking

During this phase, it is important to collect much information and news on the client's past and work on building trust. The therapist identifies the specific goals and the target memories for reprocessing. Target memories include the events that contributed to develop the pathology at first, the current originating causes that stimulate the dysfunctional material, but also the behaviours, attitudes and positive cognitions required for the future. Thus, three levels of target memories are identified for EMDR processing. They should be best processed following their natural sequence: past, present and future.

Phase 2: Preparation

The goals of the preparation phase include building a therapeutic alliance with the client, psychoeducation on trauma and the reported disorder, explaining the EMDR method and teaching relaxation techniques to manage emotions, which can be used by the client both at the end of the session and during the week to improve their own affect-regulation skills. The client must feel reassured that the work on intense discomforting emotions and on the accompanying feelings shall be performed gradually and respecting his own ability to tolerate painful experiences (Dworkin, 2005).

Phase 3: Assessment

The primary components in the traumatic memory are identified, which shall be processed with EMDR – specifically, the image that represents the worst part in the event, the associated negative cognition (an irrational negative cognition of their own self), the positive belief of their own self that the client would like to have, the emotions related to the event, the level of subjective disturbance (through the SUD – subjective unit of disturb scale) and the body position where this disturbance is felt.

Phase 4: Desensitisation

In this phase, reprocessing is performed according to some structured procedures, which involve the brain associative processes and stimulate the memory networks to guarantee that the relevant information is addressed. New insights and new memories emerge in this phase, positive emotions replace the negative ones and the memory is adaptively stored in the wider neural networks. First, the client is asked to focus on the target memory (an image, a negative belief, a feeling), and at the same time, bilateral stimulation is administered. During desensitisation, the therapist performs some BLS sets of about 30 seconds, through eye movements or other stimulation modalities, while the client focuses on some elements in the traumatic experience. After each set, the client provides a short feedback describing the perceived changes. This continues until the reported level of disturbance goes down to zero on the SUD scale. The client remains fully vigilant during the whole process; the therapist's role in this phase is to create the safety and containment conditions required to allow the client to start the reprocessing of the traumatic material by setting the best conditions for reprocessing to take place successfully. The therapist intervenes the least possible and observes the whole process with the client. The therapist can intervene actively when the reprocessing stops or is stuck to foster its reactivation.

Phase 5: Installation

This phase in the protocol focuses on strengthening the positive cognition the client has identified in Phase 3 – assessment, checking its appropriateness and validity as regards the event memory, through the VOC (validity of cognition) scale.

Phase 6: Body scan

In this phase, the client concentrates on the memory and on the positive cognition and performs a mental body examination to check the possible presence of residual disturbing physical sensations (tensions, pain, etc.), which shall be processed – if required – through later BLS sets until they disappear.

Phase 7: Closing

At the end of the session, the therapist tells the client that new memories or memory fragments could come up in the following days, including images, thoughts, physical sensations or emotions connected to the traumatic event. Thus, it is paramount to make note of all the emerged changes so that the client can talk about them with the therapist during the following session. However, the therapist remains available in case the client needs to contact him.

Phase 8: Revaluation

This phase takes place during the session after the traumatic memory has been fully reprocessed to establish any possible residual disturbance (on the SUD scale) that may still be there. This step is fundamental to ensure that the process has been completed before passing onto reprocessing the following memory.

Shapiro (2001) describes EMDR as a three-pronged protocol, in which disorders are processed starting from their antecedents, their current manifestations and their future occurrence ('future templates').

The EMDR protocol focuses on the following:

Past: unprocessed traumatic memories are stored in a state-dependent form and they are at the basis of problems, symptoms and disorders reported in the present.

Present: current situations and triggers must be specifically addressed to help the client attain a more adaptive condition in the present and, hence, a better psychological health.

Future: the memory reprocessing and integration in positive memory networks adaptively affect the client's behaviour and attitude in the future.

Thus, the work with EMDR facilitates the innate rebuilding capacity of our episodic memory. Memories (duly processed and desensitised through the work on the past) are rebuilt by putting together the more adaptive fragmented information and by increasing motivation to act and solve the problems. Based on the client's life history and the symptom organisation, case conceptualisation allows for the formulation of a therapeutic plan to process past traumatic experiences, maintain present symptoms and prepare for future challenges.

Chapter 6

EMDR applied to the treatment of individual problems

Elena Isola and Bruna Maccarrone

6.1 The EMDR protocol for individual sexual dysfunctions

The specific goal of this protocol is to define the main guidelines to treat sexual dysfunctions using the EMDR method. The conceptual framework of this protocol is the attachment theory.

6.2 Specific protocol phases to treat individual sexual dysfunctions

Phase 1: History taking

Investigate the attachment bonds with the family of origin, any traumatic experiences and/or griefs. Outline the history of the current symptom or problem (including its duration and pervasiveness). Analyse the therapeutic request (Why now?). Negative and dysfunctional cognitive schemes. Sexological assessment. Risk factors and/or possible persistence of the symptom/problem. Assessment of the client's general health condition. Identification of resources; conceptualisation and identification of target memories. Definition of the therapeutic plan.

Phase 2: Preparation

Psychoeducation; explanation of how the method works; and the therapeutic contract, resource installation and possible work on the dissociated parts of the self. In the case of the investigated protocol, additional later phases from 3 to 8 are not specifically adapted. Thus, their description remains valid as in the standard protocol.

6.2.1 Phase 1: History taking

To produce a good aetiological assumption or 'case conceptualisation', it is paramount to perform a detailed history taking on the client's life history and sexual

DOI: 10.4324/9781003508670-7

development, the history of the sexual symptom/problem and the client's current functioning. It is also relevant to define the desired therapeutic goals clearly with the client.

The client's attachment history

During history taking, it is important to obtain specific information concerning the family of origin and the attachment bond to the caregivers. Using some questions from the Adult Attachment Interview can facilitate collecting this information. This semi-structured interview is a very useful tool in clinical practice. In fact, it allows considering the client's current symptoms as a reaction to the behavioural models learnt during the first interactions with the caregivers and later strengthened through following affect relationships. The therapist can identify the emotional climate of the client's first experiences and his/her representational schemes and investigate traumatic experiences like losses, abuses, separation from the attachment figures and the current relationship with their own children. The therapist investigates the client's ability to provide a description at semantic (general knowledge, meanings, symbols and their connections) and episodic (specific information and events, their position in time and with regard to the individual's identity) levels of the relationship to reference figures by reporting the most relevant episodes specifically related to the areas of physical/emotional vulnerability. Examples include diseases or emotional difficulties, separation from the parents and feeling of rejection (Zaccagnino, 2017).

Current problem/s (including duration and seriousness; Why treatment now?)

From the first sessions, the therapist and the client together can provide meaning to the presented symptoms. It is paramount to investigate the problem the way the client represents it and assigns it with meaning. When gathering information, we must include the connection with symptoms on one side and the client's past and present experiences on the other. After analysing the problem area related to the disorder, the trigger that led to the symptom onset may be identified: the precipitating factor. You can also investigate the strategies the client has implemented to tackle the current problem and whether they have worked or not.

What painful memories does the current problem trigger in the client? If there is none, can the client simply remember or make connections to any past traumas of the same kind?

For the sake of history taking, some trigger memories can be identified through the float-back technique or starting from a bridge emotion. The client shall be asked to think about the negative cognition (float-back) or a bridge emotion and about the trigger event that the client brings into the session. By keeping both in mind, the client shall have to focus on the part of the body where he/she feels the disturbance. The next question asks when the client remembers to have felt something similar.

Sexological Assessment

The reported sexual problems are quite often just on the surface, and they hide lacking or lost relational and intimate connection behind them. For an accurate survey of the sexual history to be performed, the aspects of the client's individual functioning shall have to be investigated as regards sexuality. The dysfunctional aspects of individual sexuality will have to be analysed, including those related to couple relationships, family, social, affect and relational aspects. To this purpose, a checklist can be used to summarise the main investigation fields, which the therapist must analyse during the assessment phase and the clinical interview. The checklist is given later in detail.

Risk and/or maintenance factors

It is important to analyse all the aspects connected to sexuality in the relational field where the client has grown up and that can be considered as risk or maintenance factors of a dysfunctional behaviour. In addition, it is also paramount to analyse the modalities used by both current and past partners to relate to the client's disturbance.

The therapeutic relationship

Setting up a trust relationship is fundamental to build the therapeutic alliance, which is a must-have to attain a positive outcome for the treatment. Some major behaviours leading to create trust between the client and the therapist are the definition of the mutual roles and responsibilities and the fine-tuning on the client's needs and times.

Identification of the target memories and of a therapeutic plan

To identify the target memories for the intervention, the information collected from the client's personal history must be used, with special reference to unresolved traumas that allow connecting the current discomfort to earlier experiences.

The start is the client's present issue brought into therapy, for instance a disturbing body sensation, an unpleasant emotion, a negative cognition, or the material that keeps on emerging from the client's reports. This is used more or less systematically to try to go back to the past with the mind, wondering: 'Where does it come from? When did you experience this for the first time?' Once identified the target memories related to the client's history and the history of the sexual problem, an order of priorities should be given, to which reference can be made to structure the therapeutic plan.

Past events

Past events that have laid the foundations for the onset of the sexual dysfunction or issue may be any of the following:

- T traumas (i.e. intrusive surgery or medical examinations that concerned the genitals, harassment and sexual violence); or
- t (relational) traumas connected to the critical nucleus related to sexuality, which have structured the vulnerability that contributed to develop the disorder. For instance, you can ask the client, 'What is the first memory of sexuality you can think of?' It can be useful to explore the sentiments and feelings experienced on that occasion, and during the story telling, the therapist should check for the presence of possible traces of shame and guilt. For example, a client had always suffered from severe sexual pains, but EMDR allowed returning to an early gynaecological visit her mother obliged her to undergo when she was 9, when the doctor forced her to continue.

Present events

The work is on the body image and the memories that have contributed to generate suffering and discomfort: the first, the worst and the last time. EMDR helps the client reprocess the negative sexual experience to avoid that the negative beliefs connected to the failure become negative cognitions, fears and future situations of avoidance. For example, when a *defaillance* occurs for the first time, the client can react by tending to postpone the moment of a future sexual encounter for fear of failing again. Many clients declare 'not to be worthy as a person' or not to feel like a 'real man' after the first failures. Therapy must help the client not to perceive sex as an examination or an anxiety-triggering situation; in fact, it should instead stir passion and excitement. The correlation between the sexual symptom and the earlier negative experiences must be identified; this is quite relevant when treating sexual dysfunctions that are often accompanied by feelings of shame, guilt, humiliation and powerlessness.

In addition, since sexual reactions can be easily influenced, the negative feelings of fear, guilt or possible pain of all kinds must be reprocessed, which the client may have associated with the sexual experience, thus generating possibly inhibiting reactions.

The future model

The client is asked to imagine – in a positive and desired way – the next time he/she will be in an intimate situation to reduce anticipatory anxiety and process any possible residual memories or disturbances that may compromise current functioning. If the client reports any level of disturbance during the future projection, some BLS sets will be performed until the level of disturbance is down to zero. For example, with clients who fear having sex and who wonder whether it will happen again, it is no surprise that this concern is often accompanied by fear as an emotional state and by the client's tendency to focus on the erection, which guarantees the realisation of the prophecy.

In these situations, the work on the future template is paramount since it can break the previous negative associative chain and let new adaptive material emerge.

6.2.2   Phase 2: Preparation

Psychoeducation

The therapist must help the client understand – through psychoeducation (Dworkin, 2010) – how fundamental it is to acquire present orientation and a sense of safety inside the session. In this phase of therapy, it is paramount to provide specific indications on the male and female sexual functioning. The therapist must explain that an effective sexual intercourse depends on a complex sequence of hormonal and physiological phenomena that are extremely vulnerable to the effects of emotional excitement. Please note that fear or rage are accompanied by some deep psychological reactions that can interfere directly with the autonomously mediated vascular reflexes, which cause the erection in men and lubrication and turgidity in women. In addition, the therapist must explain that sexual reactions for men and women depend on the right hormonal balance and specifically on an appropriate measure of androgens. Moreover, stress, depression, sense of defeat or chronic conflict can cause relevant endocrine changes that reduce the circulation of androgens along the hypothalamic-pituitary axis.

The therapist must show the connection between a long-lasting negative emotional state and the onset of several psychosomatic disorders, *inter alia* sexual disorders. During psychoeducation, it is paramount to help the clients erase all forms of misinformation. For instance, the myth of simultaneous orgasm is very dangerous since many couples try to have it as if it were the only authentic goal of sexual beatitude and normality. In fact, simultaneous coital orgasms are an exception rather than the rule. A woman who bothers too much about her slower reaction can find it difficult to let herself go, and she may start enacting a constant simulation of sexual pleasure. Many women suffering from sexual problems find it important that men are satisfied first. This may depend on several factors, of both cultural (men 'must be satisfied') and emotional nature since women fear losing their partners (Vaccaro, 2003).

In this phase of psychoeducation, it is fundamental to let clients understand that the sexual reaction cannot be controlled voluntarily, that fluctuations in the sexual interest are normal and that age and life difficulties can diminish the man's sexual capacities. Alternatively, clients can react to a normal, temporary low libido or to a transient erection difficulty by showing deep, unnecessary concerns that may originate serious dysfunctional syndromes on the long run. Men over 50 years of age, who were used to obtaining a quick erection by simply touching a woman in youth, often do not understand that they must be stimulated more intensely to function normally. The anxiety originating from this and their inability to adjust to the natural slower reaction by sharing their changed needs with their partner often cause secondary impotency in midlife. A serene acceptance of the changes undergone by one's body helps propose oneself as objects of desire and of sexual initiative. Then the fundamental processes must be described accurately as regards the EMDR procedure and its working.

Resource identification and installation

By 'resources', we mean all the personal skills, abilities, belongings, relations and services that facilitate self-regulation and provide a sense of competence and resilience. Resource development starts by acknowledging and understanding the existing ones: the clients' abilities and their current competences as adults. Resource development helps clients stabilise in this phase and provides support to address and process traumatic memories in a later phase. The therapist acts as an 'auxiliary cortex' (Diamond, 1965) and as an 'affect regulator of the client's dysregulated states' to provide an environment that fosters the growth of the client's immature structures for affectivity regulation (Schore, 2001).

Emotional self-regulation and relaxation techniques

It is required to provide instructions and lessons that enable to client to learn some *emotional self-regulation and relaxation techniques*.

RESPIRATORY TRAINING

A simple, effective way to relax is to change breathing appropriately.

It is useful to ask the client how he/she breathes. In most cases, clients with these problems show short, fast breathing, with a rigid diaphragm. Diaphragmatic breathing consists in learning how to breathe according to the body's natural breathing. Some life situations or habits, in fact, can lead us to costal breathing with the following reduced air intake and the need to increase our respiratory frequency. Diaphragmatic breathing, instead, allows expanding the pulmonary basis and recovering the body's natural breathing rhythm. When seated, with the back leaning on the chair and the feet on the ground, the client is asked to put his/her open hand palms on the sides, the index fingers below the lowest anterior thoracic rib, the thumbs backwards and the remaining fingers resting on the outside margins of the upper abdominal wall. By normal breathing, the client will notice if and how much the abdomen's outer walls expand. The client will then be invited to breathe in for the air intake to push downwards and generate the abdomen's expansion.

Then the client can lay down in a comfortable position for all his/her muscles to relax. First, a deep breath-in at chest level, letting air out slowly from the mouth and slowly closing the eyes at the same time. Attention is focused on the abdomen and the tummy, and the breathing rhythm is noticed. When the clients can breathe with their tummy, they start breathing in from the nose and out from the mouth more slowly. While breathing in from the nose and out from the mouth more slowly, the client can observe what is happening to the body. The client can observe the body in full, from tiptoe to the top of the head, whether any tensions are present, or a part of the body is relaxing and if relaxation is similar to lightness or heaviness, or the body somehow tingles.

SAFE PLACE

During this exercise, the client is asked to identify a memory or a place that evokes positive sensations of safety and calmness in him/her. Later, the client is asked to focus on the feelings and emotions that he/she feels when thinking about that place and to identify where he/she can feel it in the body. The image is strengthened and short BLS sets follow. To conclude, the client is asked to think about a key word that represents the 'safe place' and the feelings associated with it, followed by some short BLS sets to strengthen all the positive emotions and associations that are coming up.

The goal of the 'safe place' exercise is to help the client become familiar with the EMDR method before the traumatic memories are processed and to provide a useful tool to reduce a possible discomfort in case the processing is not completed by the end of the session (Zaccagnino, 2017). The 'safe place' exercise helps clinicians diagnose if the client can develop an own sense of safety and understand if he/she can maintain dual attention. Furthermore, the 'safe place' allows self-modulating negative emotions.

THE 'FOUR ELEMENTS' EXERCISE FOR STRESS MANAGEMENT (ELAN SHAPIRO)

The exercise is made up by four – short and soothing – self-control activities. The 'four elements' (earth, air, water and fire) flow one after the other along the whole body, from the feet to the stomach, through the chest and the throat, up to the mouth and even higher through the head. This sequence starts from the ground to represent the safety, which lies in the present reality, and goes upwards towards the safety that is re-evoked with the help of imagination (Luber, 2015). The installation of the four elements resource and of the 'safe place' should be performed in two different sessions.

Resource installation

Three categories of resources can be developed to address the discomfort connected to male and female sexual dysfunctions:

- Mastery resources: the clients' tendency to produce negative mental images when they see the occasion of a sexual encounter inhibits the activity of their sexual circuits. To help these clients change this view and focus on the best moment in their sexual life, you can collect their most positive sexual experiences – when possible – and use one of these experiences as a 'mastery resource'. A mastery resource is the same client's memory of his/her effective management of a sexual experience and of the related positive emotions, or a physical condition or movement that imply the ability to answer to the sexual response in an effective way.

- Relational resources: the memory of a positive role example (real or taken from a book, a movie or the like) or a memory of a loving person. For instance, you can recommend buying erotic books, which are characterised by allusive atmospheres and intimacy that are not described in a straightforward way. They can be used to stimulate fantasy and let the most involving situations emerge again. Instead, if clients prefer a more explicit and direct form of eroticism, they can watch a movie with explicit sexual contents.
- Symbolic resources: the memory of an object in nature or of an archetypical or spiritual symbol or experience, a figure from their own dreams, an image taken from an artwork, a metaphor suggested by the therapist or even some music, which can evoke feelings of strength and calmness.

Identifying desires

It is important that clients can know and extend their own erotic imagery. Thus, we must identify what actually kicked off the client's sexual desires and sexual life so that – in the course of the therapeutic path – the client can express them in real life, both as a single person and within a couple. This helps the client who is facing a problematic sexual dysfunction not to blame him/herself excessively and be more self-confident towards restoring a happy sexuality. Night erotic dreams can be included herein, which have stimulated sexual fantasy particularly. The client can be asked what connection there is between the dream and the current situation, and the therapist can assess whether performing bilateral stimulation (BLS) or not. In this way, you are working on the sense of self-effectiveness and you are increasing the sense of safety and motivation to treatment.

Motivation

From our own viewpoint, the therapeutic contract – i.e. cultivating motivation and the will to work towards a change – is an ability that permeates all the therapist's interpersonal competences. It is paramount to check the motivation scale with direct questions: 'How much motivated are you to follow a path that will help you feel better from 0 to 10?' It can be useful to ask the client about what could help increase motivation to feel better or what would risk decreasing it. The alliance with the client's emotional parts and defences becomes fundamental; the earlier you understand how they function, the earlier they can be integrated into therapy.

The therapeutic contract

To structure the therapeutic work outlined in this protocol, it is paramount to understand that some clients can show ambivalence as regards their will to change. Therefore, you must understand that we could encounter a few difficulties in building the therapeutic relationship (motivation, defences and the problem of control, shame, blocks and some dissociative traits).

In some cases, when the personality structure is excessively fragmented, the therapeutic contract must be established with the client as a whole and with each one of his/her 'parts' that have been identified. In such circumstances, it is required to contact and negotiate with the most aggressive parts since the very first sessions, considering that they can endanger therapy, the client and other people (Gonzalez Vazquez, 2013). The therapeutic contract must be established fundamentally with all the client's parts, not only with the adult part that comes to therapy. Ignoring the other parts can be interpreted by the same parts as an attempt to exclude them and to make them disappear. The therapist's acceptance and neutrality towards all the client's parts allows to start a dialogue with them, by listening to their emotions and thoughts, and to start understanding them, thus feeling empathy and sharing tasks and contents (Zaccagnino, 2017).

By using different techniques, such as acting as a moderator, the therapist can help the client create a sort of internal round table and define a space for dialogue where the parts wishing to do so can go and discuss and where conflict changes into cooperation and teamwork (Gonzalez Vazquez, 2013).

The part work

As for the part work, reference is to the theory of structural dissociation of the personality (Nijenhuis & Van der Hart, 2011), which postulates the existence of two (or more) 'parts', also defined 'ego states' in the clients suffering from it: one apparently normal part (ANP) and the emotional part/s (EP) that can be several, however. The ANP is focused on everyday life and on avoiding the trauma, while the EP is focused on the traumatic memories and on defensive action systems. Please remember that it will be important to work with the emotional parts throughout the therapeutic path.

This helps the therapist both prevent therapy dropout and increase the client's awareness of their own parts and thus to manage them at best. When the client avoids these parts of their own self, he/she is simply reiterating their experiences of solitude, desires, needs, shame and fear.

When working with dissociation, it is recommended to use Fraser's 'dissociative table' technique (1991, 2003), even though with some changes, to integrate it with EMDR work: such changes mainly relate the decision to work with the parts from the viewpoint of the 'Adult Self' and the introduction of BLS (Gonzalez Vazquez, 2013). This technique consists in asking the client to imagine inviting the different parts in a meeting place. The therapist helps the 'Adult Self' acknowledge the parts through a number of questions to help the client become familiar and develop empathy with them, in an attempt to understand what they need and how he/she can take care of them. Sometimes, the EPs may not know that the past event no longer occurs. They do not know that the past 'is over' and that we are now living a different moment in time. Hence, the ANP experiences the EPs as parts the ANP wants to get rid of.

The therapist never addresses the parts directly. The therapist teaches the 'Adult Self' how to talk to them, thus defining those parameters of respect, care and consideration that have often been missing in the family environment where the client has grown up. When the adult is scared, feels shame or is unable to manage a defined situation, this means that an automatic switch has occurred and a child part has come up and cannot manage these challenges. Some people can switch to a child part as an unaware avoidance strategy, for instance, to avoid a conflict or a moment of intimacy with their own partner or in therapy to move the attention away from significant, however painful, questions.

The control part in sexual disorders

Some clients with sexual issues often show a need to control, which is expressed towards other people (hence, towards the therapist), the client's inner world and their own body too. Internally, the client can try to control his/her actions, thoughts, emotions, acts and symptoms in a rigid, however variegated, way.

An important part of therapy consists in helping the client understand that this continuous fight does not create a real control. Instead, it increases internal division and conflict and produces an even higher loss of control. Such control loss and its consequences reinforce the client's belief about the need to maintain a strict control on their own internal phenomena. As regards the outer part, the client may react to internal chaos by rigidly controlling the environment, the people he/she relates to or the therapist (Gonzalez Vazquez, 2013). The controlling part originated with a protection goal.

By telling the story of this fragile part in need of being protected by the controlling part, the therapist can trace back to the associative channels that are more directly connected to the disorder, which can be identified as target memories and, hence, treated with the standard EMDR protocol (Zaccagnino, 2017).

Shame

Shame is an essential part in traumatisation (Leskela *et al.*, 2002), and it is strictly connected to dissociation (Irwin, 1998). In general, the client finds it difficult to describe it; shame often produces a reactive, automatic withdrawal, freezing, subjection behaviours, maladaptive actions connected to self-hate and strong attack reactions sometimes. Shame is also pervasive in most chronically traumatised people. However, the client rarely starts a conversation on this subject matter since it is painful for him/her to address it in a relational context. The therapist shall then have to support the client identifying shame and talking about it. With sexually abused clients, for example, shame is in the foreground when any kind of sexual arousal occurred. The dissociated parts involved in sexual behaviour are repudiated with disgust and shame by the other ones. For this reason, the therapist must explain to the client that victims often experience sexual arousal during the abuse, and this is a normal, almost inevitable, physiological process (van der Hart et al., 2006).

A sexual abuse often triggers a sense of guilt, and shame is typical and intense. This shame entails the elimination of what has happened for the therapist; sometimes it generates dissociation and amnesia for these episodes. When fragmentation is very intense, some parts can punish the rest of the internal system or the body, which they believe are guilty for what has happened. Silvan Tomkins (see Sedgwick and Frank, 1995) and Donald Nathanson (1992) consider shame as a fundamental affect, whose goal is to block all other affects, like arousal and excessive interest, or terror and rage, if they became uncontainable and unbearable. The physical sensations of shame remind of what Stephen Porges describes as an activation of the dorsal-vagal parasympathetic system. The dorsal-vagal parasympathetic reaction involves a reduction in the body activity, in physical energy and in breathing. When the child's early experiences include frequent examples of these 'stops' of the dorsal-vagal parasympathetic system, it is very likely that the thoughts the client formulates on their own are shaped by self-criticism as the main affect (Knipe, 2017). The therapist should not deny the client's shame experience so neatly, but he/she should empathise with it and help the client verbalise and explore it (Nathanson, 1992).

The 'loving eyes' procedure

The 'loving eyes' procedure consists in asking one part, usually the ANP, to shape a visual picture of an EP, usually a younger part that is reliving a traumatic event. A phobic fear usually characterises the relationship between these two parts (van der Hart et al., 2006). An ANP can have phobic attitudes towards an EP due to the EP's overwhelming content, for fear of the disruptive influence the EP could exert on the ANP's main function, i.e. fulfilling the everyday life tasks the ANP must perform and maintaining an apparent normality in the meantime. In addition, EPs are often scared by the simple thought that they have to confront with the ANP's judgment. The ANP is often phobic and scared not only by the EPs but also by particular memories and specific actions that have something to do with the trauma (like rage, sexual activation, the need for nourishment and sometimes the fear of the same fear) too. Strong avoidance defences may have already been enacted, possibly in a non-conscious way, if they are experienced as a need to be able to defend oneself by maintaining a dissociative split between the parts. Some BLS sets can be used for this type of problem to start the resolution of the internal conflict that was unresolvable at the beginning. By defining appropriate target memories for reprocessing, the parts can become mutually more aware. They can be helped – thanks to the 'loving eyes' procedures – to be less scared of one another. The internal dialogue driven by the therapist can even soften the mutual oppositions (Knipe, 2017).

An essential element in a healthy attachment style between children and caretakers is a good mutual eye contact, which is mutually pleasant and soothing (Schore, 2002). Eye contact is essential for connection. The 'loving eyes' procedure is a way to help clients develop – one step after another – this type of soothing connection, whose result is a conversation between the parts that were dissociative and conflicting at the beginning. It is particularly useful in two opposed situations: when fear (rage or despair) is too strong and makes it impossible to create a direct contact between the parts and when, at the beginning, the mutual affect communication is too low due to the excessive dissociative distance between the parts.

The use of drawings

Drawings can shape the traumatic aspects connected to sexual issues, the related fears and their own relationship with them.

Drawings can help the client be safe and stable, which allows him to access the destabilising world of the traumatic experience without losing their own balance.

When clients start to feel disoriented upon their acknowledging a system of parts within them, the possibility to represent the different parts on a single sheet of paper provides them with containment and control. The method simply consists in asking the client to draw a 'map' showing the relevant information on their own internal experience: 'Can you draw something to represent the experience you are living now, in this very moment?' The 'map' can be a representation of all the known elements in the client's personality structure, or it can be an image to represent the parts involved in the memory of a specific emotionally-laden event (Knipe, 2017).

6.3 Application of the EMDR protocol to individual therapy

Mario's case

The client is a young man aged 30 who works as a graphic designer in a large company. He lives alone, and he is apparently shy, introverted and controlled. He asks for help because he is worried about the sexual symptom he is experiencing during intercourses with the girl he is going out with. The relationship he is having now started about six months ago, and it is his first stable relationship in which he feels involved. A clear difficulty emerges to confront freely with the female world and to open up to a sexual relationship without fears. Mario met B. (aged 27) thanks to some common friends. He does not tell her he has decided to start a sexological path; he does not feel their relationship is stable enough, and in addition, she lives in a different city. The week before calling to start therapy, Mario had his first and only panic attack while he was on the train on his way back to his hometown. When trying to narrate the events, Mario says that the evening before, he had slept with B. for the first time and that he had never felt so close to a woman. The *trigger* emerging from these first encounters is his growing involvement with his partner.

The sexological assessment

During the first interviews, Mario says he feels unable and inappropriate in the sexual sphere and that he perceives his girlfriend's more experience as inhibiting. The assessment questions reveal an inappropriate sexual education: his father had never been a good counterpart on these questions, showing embarrassment when talking about them. His mother was very introverted and avoidant as regards intimate questions, however, very much focused on her son's school performance and on household organisation. When he was about 13, Mario had his first masturbation experiences, perceiving discomfort and pain to the penis and the glans during erection. Only after two years, Mario talked about this difficulty to his parents, and after an andrology check-up when he was 16, he underwent phimosis surgery and he has been very shy since then; he did not talk about this issue with his peers, and this added up to his scarce information on sexuality. With regret, Mario says he could not even integrate with his schoolmates. Before meeting B., he had had two short relationships – both lasting about three months – with no sexual intercourse.

The first diagnostic interviews showed that Mario suffered from *primary early ejaculation*, and this symptom has always been present since his first sexual intercourses, *generalised* and total because present in all the situations and independently upon the received sexual stimulus.

First assessment phase

During the following interviews, a number of elements must be further investigated in the area of development (quality and difficulties connected to the attachment history), precipitating factors (anxiety, sense of inappropriateness) and maintenance factors (inappropriate information on sexuality, conception of their own body, lacking self-esteem, performance anxiety). At the same time, an andrology check-up is recommended for an organic assessment.

Andrology history

Based on a genital check-up, an objective examination and a general medical assessment, no specific disorders emerge. In addition, a prostate control and a urethral swab were performed with standard results. The andrologist performed an assessment of the perception and knowledge of the pelvic floor muscles where, instead, a command inversion emerged. The andrologist recommended starting some Kegel exercises later on.

Individual treatment: Phase 1 in the EMDR protocol

We collected information on Mario's life history, with special focus on his attachment history and sexuality. The goal was to gain the required information to produce a good case conceptualisation and structure the therapeutic plan then.

Family history and attachment relationships

The family is made up by mother (aged 60), a housewife and father (aged 65), an engineer. Mother is very devoted to her family, very demanding, rigid and little loving. Her caretaking merely applies to the concrete organisation of family life. Father is a silent man, devoted to his job and often absent. As concerns the relationships to his parents, an attachment history progressively emerges, which is characterised by emotional neglect and an early drive to autonomy. Father took little care of him; he was often absent due to long business trips abroad. Mario's history shows a non-affective and rigid family environment, an issue of defectiveness and no lovability. To guarantee affect closeness, Mario learnt not to disregard the other's requests, not to create any problems and particularly not to ask for help so that he did not bother anyone. Mario has always been independent. He used to do his homework by himself, with no one there to control where he went, with whom and at what time he was back. The analyses of his life history allowed us to obtain the target memories that contributed to Mario's evident attachment disorganisation.

Resource identification

In addition to the aspects connected to the pathogenesis, Phase 1 in the treatment focuses on the identification of the resources that will have to be strengthened to make the later processing of traumatic events and the therapeutic change easier. In his list of ten positive memories, Mario gives some moments in his sports activity when he obtained excellent results. From 7 to 15 years of age, Mario had attended a swimming course, and he often won the year-end competitions. In addition, he remembers with pleasure the alliance with his swimming trainer. Moreover, Mario smiles when he thinks about the feel of 'diving' and the possibility to play with his peers in those moments.

Identification of the target memories and the therapeutic plan

At the end of the consultation phase, Mario is proposed a psychotherapeutic path using EMDR, which is aimed at reprocessing the most important target memories and at solving his affect difficulties with women, including his inability to live a serene and gratifying sexual life now. Mario welcomes the proposal to work on this goal with favour.

Clients with sexual symptoms sometimes find it helpful to integrate a pharmacological treatment too. In this case, given the client's young age and inexperience, and considering the clear connection between his fear for intimacy and the attachment issues, EMDR therapy only was deemed appropriate to work on the most significant target memories connected to the symptoms. The EMDR protocol for performance anxiety would be applied later. During the sessions, the connections between his painful past experiences and his current difficulties appeared more and more evidently; thus, Mario became strongly aware that old sufferings needed to be reprocessed to solve current problems.

Past events

As concerns past target memories, the following are the most important ones.

A meaningful target memory is that related to his father's long business trip abroad when Mario was 6. He remembered that his father had left during the night and that he had not found him when waking up in the morning. Mario remembered his mother's distraction when he had asked for her help. She used to remain imperturbable. Sadness and a deep sense of void emerged. Another memory dated back to when Mario was 7: he used to arrive at school by bus and see his schoolmates' parents outside the school. A third critical memory referred to when he was 8: his father had confessed to him that they had never wanted a child and his birth had been a problem. Puberty left a mark on Mario: during his first masturbation experiences, he started to have moments of anxiety and anguish. The pain perceived during erection and the difficulties to talk about that let shame and solitude emerge. In addition, Mario remembered his embarrassment and feeling different from his peers who used to joke at him when they saw his reaction at their sexual hints. Another critical episode emerged through a float-back, starting from the negative cognition 'I am defective': during a phone call, his mother had laughed and told her friend that her son was not able to masturbate. A 'big' T trauma occurred in high-school years: Mario underwent phimosis surgery when he was 15. He had not been informed about the surgery; his mother had hastily accompanied him to the hospital, and he thought it was just a check-up. His experienced rage was connected to the period of his penis surgery. Since his mother did not know how to manage the situation, she talked about her son's difficulties with everyone, thus provoking Mario's deep shame. This experience was disorganising since he was exposed to judgment, and his mother neither contained nor protected him against the experienced shame and humiliation.

Present events (trigger events)

- I worked on body image and symptom on all the most recent events connected to Mario's negative beliefs, which contributed to creating suffering and discomfort, processing the first, the worst and the last times when he suffered a sexual dysfunction.
- I worked on the panic attack following his *defaillance*.

Future template

- The next time, he will feel affectively involved with his partner.
- The next time, he will have to express what he needs.
- The next time, he will complete sexual intercourse.

These are the most significant target memories addressed in the initial phase of treatment even if later on – as it often happens with EMDR – new memory networks can reactivate, with other memories emerging connected to the problem. In such case, the therapeutic plan shall be reviewed and renegotiated regarding the newly emerged memories.

Phase 2: the client's preparation

To prepare Mario for the following processing work on traumatic memories, specific information is provided concerning EMDR therapy: how eye movements and other forms of alternated bilateral stimulation work, how the innate information processing mechanism works and the impact of traumatic events on how our personality develops in addition to later possible problems.

Before starting reprocessing traumatic memories, it was appropriate to strengthen and stabilise Mario's personality through some techniques to install and strengthen his resources. This allows establishing an internal 'safe base' that fosters the potential resilience and strengthens coping abilities too.

Resource installation

Before processing target memories with EMDR, Mario completed four sessions to develop and install resources with the RDI (Resource Development Installation) protocol to foster higher initial stabilisation and enhance affect regulation and coping abilities (Korn and Leeds, 2002; Leeds and Shapiro, 2000). Then some psychoeducational sessions and 35 EMDR sessions were held within about nine months.

The first installed resource, namely, the 'safe place', was aimed at eliciting a sense of calmness and safety. Then other resources were identified to help Mario address his current difficulties. Mario reported that the positive personal qualities that would be helpful included enhancing his assertiveness in interpersonal relationships and, specifically, being able to communicate his needs and feelings. During the RDI sessions, Mario was asked to focus on his own specific autobiographical positive memories when he felt he had had the desired qualities and resources, which – however – were in no way associated with those negative memories that would be later processed. Following the RDI protocol steps, the perception of a competent and appropriate adult state and the related feelings were installed and strengthened. The identified resource concerned a memory of when he had won a swimming competition and his trainer had hold him in his arms with affection.

EMDR sessions

The standard EMDR protocol from Phase 3 to 8 was applied to every target memory identified during the history taking phase.

The first part of therapy focused on processing all those early memories regarding the attachment relationships that had had a traumatic impact on the development of Mario's personality, thus defining a vulnerable structure and a critical inappropriateness nucleus in him, which later reflected on his sexuality. All these events were processed in chronological order according to the AIP model and following the past-present-future template. Mario was worried because of his partner's request to bring their connection to a deeper level, and he felt this pressure would jeopardise the identity he had built with much effort throughout the years, based on self-sufficiency and the capacity to be enough for himself. The first EMDR sessions focused on the reprocessing of memories related to attachment traumas and showed deep solitude and affective neglect in Mario's past. One of the target memories reporting a very high SUD referred to an event when he was 8: his father had told him that they had never wanted to have any children. This session was very laden with emotions: Mario could express intensely his pain and the emotions connected to the refusal he had perceived in his father's narrative. At a certain point, he saw himself 'alone' in the memory; however, discomfort started to diminish.

Thanks to the processing of the past events, Mario strengthened his awareness of the connection between current difficulties and past-related events. He acknowledged the regulatory function of the sexual symptom that he used to address his sense of inappropriateness and his anxiety and fear states before treatment. The second part of the therapy focused on the disorder, the symptoms and the connected memories, always in chronological order and following the past-present-future template. The following EMDR sessions focused on reprocessing the memories related to the phimosis surgery since his parents had not prepared him, and instead, they had told him that it was to be a normal check-up.

While continuing the reprocessing of the various target memories linked to the hospitalisation issue, Mario acknowledged that his guilt and shame for the experienced exposure were being progressively replaced by growing anger. After closing the processing of the memory when he had felt a nurse was joking at him, other memories emerged, mainly related to his mother's neglecting behaviour: 'I had never thought I had not been protected'.

During his last sexual intercourse with his partner, Mario had experienced strong discomfort, and he understood he tended to skip foreplay and not to take the sexual initiative. Starting from the worst image of the last intercourse, from the negative cognition and the localisation of the disturbance in the body, Mario was able to connect his strong emotional discomfort to the hand-genitals contact linked to a check-up after his surgery. In such sense, the body had played a fundamental role in reactivating his traumatic memories.

Therapy closing

Mario arrived for a new session saying he had perceived higher assertiveness in his behaviour compared to the past, which allowed him to live sex with his partner with less fear and passivity. Answering a comment on his early ejaculation, he was able to answer appropriately, and he did not to feel threatened. Mario started relying on the possibility of leaving his difficulties behind, and his friends and current partner noticed that he was more serene. During the following sessions, he confirmed his progress in the relationship with his partner and reported that they had booked a holiday together. They were also living sexual intimacy in a more serene way. Mario told me that they had both started allowing more time for fore-play and they had experienced their best and most satisfactory coital intercourse up to that moment. At the same time, with the help of the sexual tasks, Mario had become more aware of his body and increased his level of relaxation during sexuality. To this purpose, Kegel exercises were particularly useful, as recommended by the andrologist after highlighting the command inversion at the level of the muscles in the pelvic floor.

Post-treatment outcome

A CHANGE IN THE SEXUAL SYMPTOM

Mario no longer meets the generalised early ejaculation disorder criteria. The discovery of pleasant sensations without the burdening comparative/examination feeling allowed him to increase his control over his ejaculation, which is now quite satisfactory. He is currently showing a good mood; he addresses sexual intercourses with growing serenity, and he feels he is progressively getting closer to his partner. During the follow-up after six months, he confirmed full remission from his symptom.

CHANGES IN THE ATTACHMENT STYLE

The administration of the AAI (Adult Attachment Interview) after the EMDR treatment showed increased safety and an evolution towards a safer attachment style. Mario has reduced his negative beliefs related to self-esteem and vulnerability thanks to the EMDR reprocessing of previous relational memories.

RELATION WITH THE SELF

The goal was to change the negative cognition of inadequacy and the following sense of self-defectiveness. After treatment, Mario showed higher self-acceptance.

AFFECT REGULATION

The goal was to increase Mario's ability to recognise, express and regulate his emotions as regards sexuality.

CHANGES IN EVERYDAY LIFE

Mario increased his social skills, which have brought him to better interactions with his peers and higher assertiveness in his interactions with his partner searching for more situations that are social.

Discussion

At the beginning of his path, the client was unable to provide a consistent narrative; events were somehow disconnected. The narrated episodes were painful for Mario; however, they were not perceived as if they were mutually related. Particularly, the client was not able to relate his life history to his reported symptom. Personifying the occurred events has given him the possibility to contact the child who had never been able to express himself before and to tell his fears and sense of inadequacy. Providing meaning to his own discomfort, understanding the reason for his disorder and connecting it to his own life history enabled the processing and change in the self-referred negative cognitions. Today, Mario no longer perceives himself as 'not lovable'. Now he feels 'worthy of being loved'. Working on the unresolved nuclei of the attachment relations has allowed us to access work on the present and the future now, with the goal to help Mario recover a good level of affect and sexual intimacy.

EMDR can really help the client help himself so that he can help the child who experienced the traumatic events to let repressed memories emerge and be expressed. This also allows changing the internal working models related to the client's attachment history by not only dealing with what happened but also with what did not happen unfortunately. From one point of view, in fact, such therapeutic approach represents the attempt to intervene on the client's attachment history.

The therapeutic relationship stirred sadness, anger, shame and powerlessness, and the therapist and the client experienced some intense moments of connection building. Therapy ended when Mario gained an internal sense of consistency and wholeness, and he was able to take up his present and plan his future.

Please note that the names chosen for the narrative of the mentioned clinical cases are invented to protect the clients' privacy.

6.4   Checklist for the individual sexological assessment

With reference to the sexological assessment mentioned in Phase 1, here follows a checklist with the main fields for investigation that the therapist must analyse during the clinical interview.

1. Problem definition.
2. Physical health (with possible in-depth medical examinations, where required, particularly in case of erection disorders).
3. List of any drugs possibly taken.
4. The family's attitudes and education as concerns sexuality: communication modalities, tackling nakedness at home, pre-marriage sexual activity, masturbation, homosexuality, etc.
5. Modalities to learn the main facts about sexuality and reproduction (including the changes that occur during puberty, menstruation, nocturnal emissions) from parents, teachers, peers, etc.

6. Any religious beliefs on sexuality (masturbation, petting, pre-marriage sex, abortion, contraception, etc.).

7. Beliefs related to specific aspects of sexuality: distinction of sexual roles when taking the sexual initiative (for instance, the conviction that the man must always do that); the importance assigned to the penis size with reference to the ability to produce pleasure in a woman; the (wrong) conviction according to which once a man has his erection, this remains unaltered throughout the whole sexual intercourse (alternatively, it means that there are some problems for the man, or the woman does not arouse him enough); the belief that the climax must necessarily be reached during the sexual intercourse or however following penetration; any attitudes regarding oral or anal practices, etc.; the (wrong) belief that simultaneous climax is the best and 'correct' way to attain sexual satisfaction.

8. Beliefs on the distinctions between male and female sexual roles. Presence of possible 'double standards'.

9. Stories of past sexual and/or affect experiences and of sexual satisfaction with reference to them.

10. The story of a possible current affect/sexual connection and of past and present sexual satisfaction with the current partner.

11. Modalities to have a climax: alone, with the partner, vaginal or clitoral orgasm.

12. Satisfaction related to the frequency and quality of their own climax. Comparison with the satisfaction about its frequency and quality in past sexual experiences with other partners and with the current one. Possible dissatisfaction in case no orgasm is possibly attained during the sexual intercourse (analysing the reactions, whether the unattained climax is their own or the partner's).

13. Need that orgasm is attained through penetration or acceptance of the fact that it can be reached through other modalities (or in a way by one partner and in a different way by the other). Need to have a climax for the sexual intercourse to be deemed satisfactory.

14. It is important to be able to bring the partner to feel pleasure. Need to notice that you have produced pleasure for the partner before being able to attain it.

15. Possible current masturbatory practices (sexual activity without a partner) and satisfaction or dissatisfaction related to them. Attitude towards masturbation – even in adulthood – if there is a sexual partner. Possible sense of guilt related to masturbation, both past and present.

16. Satisfaction about the frequency of sexual encounters with the partner or others.

17. In general, is there any communication with the partner or others about the sexual sphere?

18. Are there any erotic fantasies? When? How often? Are they a source of excitement? Of discomfort? Are they approved?

19. Are there any dreams with sexual contents? How often?

20. Do you feel discomfort with your naked body? Why? When?

21. How satisfied are you with your body?

22. Do you think you are physically attractive for your partner?

23. Any used contraceptive methods and level of satisfaction for them.
24. Attitudes and beliefs as regards homosexuality.
25. Have you ever felt sexual attraction for same-sex people? Does this bother you?
26. Possible use of external tools for sexual excitement: readings, magazines, videos, alcohol, drugs, couple exchange, group sex, etc. Are these practices shared with the partner or friends too?
27. Possible paraphilic sexual excitement (this area needs to be investigated with special caution since it could not be declared spontaneously given the paraphilics' egosintonicity).
28. Assessment of their own sexual desire on a scale from 0 (absent) to 10 (extremely high).
29. Assessment of the climax intensity on a scale from 0 (absent) to 10 (extremely high).
30. Assessment of their own sexual satisfaction on a scale from 0 (absent) to 10 (extremely high).

Chapter 7

Application of EMDR in the treatment of couple's issues

Elena Isola

7.1 The EMDR protocol for couple's dysfunctions

EMDR has been applied to couple therapy in the form of both parallel individual treatment and jointly with both partners attending (Moses, 2002; Protinsky *et al.*, 2001; Shapiro, 1995).

Protinsky *et al.* (2001) reported that couples under joint EMDR treatment benefitted from 'greater emotional experiences' and observed that EMDR as a joint couple intervention seemed to enhance therapeutic effectiveness. Joint couple therapy with EMDR increases empathy in the assisting partner while the partner who is working in the session softens his/her reactivity to the events that trigger relational attachment traumas (Moses, 2002).

Johnson and Whiffen (2003) suggested that couple therapy could offer alternative models to respond and new ways to relate to each other. Strengthening the couple's bond offers relational resilience and mutual emotional protection (Shapiro and Laliotis, 2011).

Working together balances the system since no partner is identified as the 'problem' and both can access past wounds while the partner is assisting in a compassionate way, thus experimenting pain vicariously and activating mutual fine-tuning. This increase in empathy and understanding can accelerate a fundamental shift since old, tough, disturbing narratives are replaced by new, more tender and loving stories. The reduction in the emotional load of past experiences allows the couple to respond without reactivity, with less stress on the past and more energy on present interactions. Thus, treatment works a system correction (Shapiro and Laliotis, 2011). Holmes (1998) highlighted that the awareness of the other's unmet primary attachment needs encourages acceptance of the fact that he/she is not acting in 'a deliberately contrary way; however, the partner is pursuing some models that operate unconsciously'.

Therapists are recommended to apply EMDR jointly only after they have checked for the partners' commitment, safety and mutual consent. Joint EMDR is not recommended in case of serious trauma or reluctance, hostility or intolerance by one partner due to the implied emotional intensity (Shapiro and Laliotis, 2011).

DOI: 10.4324/9781003508670-8

EMDR and the systemic view seem ready for a functional integration for the following reasons: one addresses the reprocessing of traumas and facilitates their desensitisation through the associated memories, which will inevitably tackle the relational contexts that have triggered and allowed them. The other focuses on trauma-generating contexts to analyse, highlight and later reprocess the dynamics that have allowed them.

7.2   Integrated sex therapy

Integrated sex therapy can be both individual and with the couple. It offers a number of prescriptions in terms of sexual behaviours or 'tasks', whose goal is to work on four specific areas involved in sexuality, depending on the clinician's initial assessment, i.e.:

1. Knowledge of their own self. It relates to the personal and behavioural knowledge of their own body and sexual responses starting from visual and tactile exploration: the exploration of thoughts, internal dialogue and imaginary and emotional content obtained through self-observation.
2. Knowledge of their own self with the other. The partner becomes a mirror where you can observe yourself at three levels:

   • The behavioural one, with reference to the partner's body and sexual responses;
   • The cognitive one, intended as the discovery of the partner's emotional response and desires; and
   • The relational one.

3. The knowledge of their own pleasure and experiences: the possibility to experience sexual pleasure, to discover it in its individual aspects and to contact their own emotions.
4. The knowledge of the couple's intimacy: the exploration of useful behaviours to attain mutual pleasure and the exposure to growing levels of intimacy by sharing sexual emotions to experience mutual trust as a goal in a cooperation process.

Sensory focus I

The couple is asked not to have sexual intercourse and climax for several days and weeks. During this period, however, the partners are asked to caress each other's body and genitals tenderly. This can be prescribed only when the nature of the dysfunction and the needs in the dynamic of that specific case seem to require it. For instance, it can be prescribed to a couple if the two partners are too fixated on the climax or if they must tackle the anxiety they feel when they are in intimacy. It can also be prescribed when working with a partner who has erective difficulties due to women's general lack of reaction and related climax inhibitions. The prescription of 'sensory focus I' often produces a reduction in tension during sexual intercourses. Each partner is freed from the expectation according to which he/she must trigger an appropriate reaction in themselves or in the partner. Anticipatory anxiety connected to the idea to fail can be gradually reduced.

Sensory focus II

'Sensory focus II' is usually the step following 'sensory focus I'. However, treatment can start by assigning this task first in some cases. In 'sensory focus II', the partners are asked to mutually stimulate the genitals in turns, with the goal to trigger excitement but not the orgasm. If a couple reports they have experienced negative feelings – for instance, if it is guilt because they are feeling and showing pleasure openly, or hidden hostility against the partner, or the fear to be rejected – the therapist shall work on trying to tackle this difficulty.

7.3   The EMDR protocol to treat sexual issues in the couple and specific phases for the treatment of sexual dysfunctions in the couple

The specific goal of this protocol is to define the main guidelines to treat sexual dysfunctions using the EMDR method. Particularly, we are focusing on the first two phases in the protocol, which are paramount to organise the following therapeutic work.

Phase 1: Individual and couple history taking

History taking shall relate to the individual's and the couple's story, the attachment bonds to the families of origin, any traumatic experiences and/or griefs, the couple's functioning and the current problem/s (including the duration and extent of the problem and why therapy is now asked for) at the basis of the intervention request. The sexological assessment will follow, with the assessment of risk and/ or maintenance factors, resource identification and the identification of the target memories required for the structuring of the therapeutic plan.

Phase 2: Preparation

Psychoeducation, explanation of the method, therapeutic contract, resource installation and work on the parts.

Phase 3: Assessment
Phase 4: Desensitisation
Phase 5: Installation
Phase 6: Body scan
Phase 7: Closing
Phase 8: Revaluation

Phase 1: Individual and couple history taking

In this phase, the therapist shall investigate the individual shared request for couple therapy and the possible absence of a therapy request by one of the two partners. The therapist shall investigate the reasons leading the couple to therapy and the modalities leading the couple to ask for help. The therapist must foster mutual listening and the definition of the individual goals for both partners. For therapy to be successful, it is paramount to obtain consent and mutual commitment after identifying the shared goals. In this phase, it is important to form a therapeutic alliance with each partner. The meetings to assess the problems brought in by the couples must be conducted both with the couple and individually. The assessment phase shall include a few meetings with the couple and other individual meetings for the partners to investigate their sexual issues in a confidential way. During the last assessment meeting, the therapist summarises what has emerged since the first session, explaining the issues referred by the couple and proposing a treatment plan.

The first phase of the EMDR treatment consists in taking up history information and news connected to the partners' personal stories, the couple's story and their sexual story. This allows performing a good initial assessment of both personal and interpersonal dynamics.

Attachment style

For an in-depth investigation of each partner's attachment history, the therapist can ask a few questions from the Adult Attachment Interview (George *et al.*, 1985), a semi-structured interview to assess the representations in adulthood of the first attachment relationships (Hesse, 1999). The questions investigate the client's ability to provide a semantic description (general knowledge, meanings, symbols and their relationships) and an episodic description (specific information and events in time and in connection with the individual's identity) of the relationship with the reference figures. This takes place through the narration of meaningful episodes specifically related to the areas of physical/emotional vulnerability, i.e. emotional difficulties or diseases, the separation from the parents, the feeling of rejection.

The therapist also asks questions to help the client reflect on the impact that early attachment relationships have had on the adult personality, such as the experiences that could represent an obstacle to growth and, to conclude, an explanation of the reasons, which – in the client's opinion – could trigger the parents' behaviour towards him/her. A section is devoted to the detailed summary of the griefs and episodes that the client considers traumatic (Zaccagnino, 2017). How does the partners' attachment style interfere with the relationship?

The partners need to be helped to become aware of how the interaction with their attachment figures could have originated some internal working models that have turned into affect-regulation strategies (Schore, 2003) and into strategies for relational interaction and how these models interact within the couple's relationship. It is important for both partners to separate the past from the present and to identify repetitive schemes. For example, a partner who has learnt to feel of little importance in his/her attachment history will perceive the same child experience and will re-enact an old story.

The couple's history

To explore the couple's history, questions are asked to understand how the relationship started, the moment when they met and the comparison with parenting model couples. The therapist analyses the couple's evolutionary phase and the extended family system.

Can the partners count on a social network, both as a couple and as individuals? Are there any conflicts with one or both families of origin? It can be useful to ask both partners to represent a timeline to identify the most meaningful positive and negative events experienced since the moment they met to their request for therapy.

The couple's functioning

Sternberg (1986a, 986b) drew up a triangular theory of love, defining it as the combination of three components to be applied to the couple and identifying different love triangles for the very same relationship. The triangles have three sides: intimacy, passion and commitment. They differ by size (the quantity of love), shape (the balance of love), the fact that they represent what we have (the real relationship) or what we would like to have (the ideal relationship) and the fact that they represent our own feelings or actions.

INTIMACY

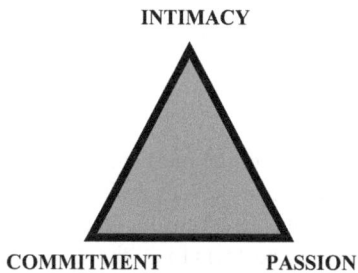

COMMITMENT   **PASSION**

The Triangular Theory of Love (Sternberg, 1986)

Commitment

The 'decision/commitment' component has two aspects: decision (short-term) is the first, and it consists in deciding to love someone; commitment (long-term) consists in maintaining the relationship in time. The two aspects can be separated since commitment does not always follow decision, and again, commitment is not always a consequence of decision.

The first issue to discuss with the partners is their definition of commitment. Do they share the same definition? Are they committed, not committed, ambivalent or committed in a different way? We believe that one of the major factors in a successful couple's therapy is commitment. When a couple comes to therapy and both partners say they are equally committed in the couple's relationship, we quite often have a couple in front of us that will manage to solve the problems they have. When the couple is ambivalent, the partners show different levels of commitment, or they seem like they do not want to commit. Here, an open discussion is required to understand thoughts and feelings in both partners.

The goal is to obtain enough long-lasting commitment towards treatment to allow for an analysis of the relationship: the couple will thus be able to check if it is possible to recover their married life or if a separation is necessary. When the partners cannot commit mutually, it is required that they commit to the therapeutic process.

Intimacy

For Sternberg (1986), intimacy means feeling close, united and connected. It means to wish the best for the other, to be concerned about the other, to speak a common language, to provide mutual emotional support and to respect and trust the other. The 'intimacy' component refers to trust, compatibility and sharing. This component defines the couple's tendency to take care of the other, to understand and accept mutually through an open and confidential communication.

After shortly describing the concept of intimacy, the therapist should explain that different individuals and different couples define intimacy in their own way; hence, ask both partners to give their definition of intimacy in their own words and later discuss about it in depth.

Passion

The 'passion' component relates to the most impulsive aspects that can characterise a love story: physical attraction, sexual desire, desire of belonging and strong emotional involvement towards the other too. Once again, the point is to describe this concept briefly and ask the partners to do the same.

STRATEGIES FOR THE COUPLE'S AFFECT REGULATION

It is important to understand deeply how the partners relate to each other when a conflict arises. To frame their modality, for instance, it can be useful to ask them to stop and reflect on some episodes of when they felt they had lost control.

'What happened? What are your partner's typical behaviours, words and expressions that activate these dysregulated responses? Are there any behaviours, words or facial expressions that make you feel humiliated, inferior, subdued?

What are the emotions you feel in these contexts? How do you feel after these reactions?'

'Do you think these interactions are the only way for you to perceive more emotional closeness?'

'Have you ever thought if it is easier for you to lose control in those moments when you feel powerless?'

Or using a float-back on the negative cognitions ('I am powerless', 'I have no control', 'I am dangerous') and/or the associated sensations/emotions:

'Again, thinking about the moments when you lose control, was there anyone in your family who could not control him/herself? Which parent used to lose control more easily? How did the other parent react in that moment? And you?'

'Can you tell me if you experience the moments of control loss with frustration and shame or humiliation? If so, try to think about what child experience triggered the same feelings in you'.

Use the emotional bridge technique:

Let's see if there are any typical signals in the body that can clearly indicate a difficulty in regulating affects. [. . .] Focus on a moment, focus on that body sensation and try to think about other moments in your life when you felt it, going back in time, possibly to your first twelve years of life (Verardo and Lauretti, 2017).

CURRENT PROBLEM/S (INCLUDING DURATION AND SERIOUSNESS OF THE PROBLEM; WHY TREATMENT NOW?)

One partner or both have a symptom that is reflected onto the couple. The disorder can be attributed to specific previous events, i.e. negative sexual experiences, sexual abuses, strict education, psychosexual difficulties or recent traumatic events (miscarriage, betrayal). Couple's therapy must help the partners understand what trigger events caused their discomfort or triggered the symptoms.

Trigger events are current situations or stimuli that activate past attachment traumas and wounds, thus defining a sort of 'coaction to reiterate'. The triggers can trigger again emotions, physiological responses and negative beliefs that can be associated with the original wound. Since these blocking behaviours and beliefs destroy the intimate relationship, it will be necessary to help the couple fight their tendency.

RISK AND/OR MAINTENANCE FACTORS

The sexual issue can become a relational strategy, and it can be used to test how strong the partner's love is. Both partners can use the symptom to avoid addressing the marital discomfort and redefine the relationship, i.e. when moving from being a couple to being a family with children. Sometimes, when one partner's sexual symptoms integrate with the other partner's ones, mutual understanding arises in the couple, and the sexual distance can become a defence against excessive intimacy.

IDENTIFICATION OF THE INDIVIDUAL'S AND COUPLE'S RESOURCES

Resources are those skills, abilities and strategies that the individual enacts to tackle and solve problems and that create a sense of self-effectiveness together with the positive feeling perceived by attaining the goal.

Just like in individual therapy, in couple's therapy, it is also important to identify individual resources. However, in addition to this, it is paramount to identify 'the couple's resources', too, i.e. the positive and constructive potential in the dyad, where individual resources are put to serve the couple, thus strengthening their resilience and ability to address marital, parenting and individual challenges. Identifying the client's functioning parts means finding an ally for the later therapeutic work. This is even more true for the couple, where it is particularly useful for therapy to identify the moments when the couple functioned well, to recover – however partially – a positive perception of the relationship. This enhances the alliance in the couple, reducing or softening the level and perception of their conflicts, and it improves the therapeutic alliance, too, by limiting the attempts to triangulate with the therapist and, hence, to boycott therapy.

This all fosters stabilisation and the preparation for the following reprocessing work on the individual's and the couple's wounds.

SEXOLOGICAL ASSESSMENT

The reported sexual problems are quite often only the facade behind which lacking or lost relational and intimate connection hides. An accurate survey of the partners' sexual history shall explore the aspects of each partner's individual functioning and of the couple's sexuality. It will include the dysfunctional aspects in the individual's and the couple's sexuality and the family, social, affective and relational aspects. To this purpose, a summary checklist can be used with the main investigation fields that the therapist must analyse during the assessment phase in the clinical interview. The checklist is reported here later.

During the sessions, attention shall be paid to the individual sensitivity as regards the experiences and the creation of meanings that the person experiences on sexuality. It is paramount to understand deeply the modality that the couple applies to experience sexuality by asking specific questions with the goal to investigate how their sexual relationship was before the symptom appeared:

'Who takes the initiative?'
'Does the sexual act originate from particular moments of sexual and/or relational understanding?'
'Describe the situations you consider supportive to the sexual act'.

'Do you feel safe when you are in sexual intimacy with your partner?'

'Do you think you have control during intimacy?'

'What makes you feel that you have no control, and what are the consequences you observe?'

'Which of your partner's behaviours tends to reduce or annihilates your sexual desire?'

'What has changed in the relationship since the symptom appeared?'

IDENTIFICATION OF TARGET MEMORIES AND THE THERAPEUTIC PLAN

Sharing the history of their families of origin with the two partners can be very useful, and it can foster understanding of how their sexual issue developed. The symptom can be defined as an opportunity for growth, which allows the couple to dedicate some time to reflect on their personal history and on how to valorise the couple. Taking care of the affect bond helps build a good relational intimacy. Some changes at individual and couple's level could help recover more psychophysical well-being. Once the personal histories are taken, the target memories are identified, which are related to the partners' history and the history of their sexual issue, which lie at the basis of the onset and maintenance of the couple's issue. For the sake of structuring the therapeutic plan, it is also quite important to identify the trigger event that altered their relationship and originated the couple's/sexual problem.

- Identification of the event triggering the disorder.
- T traumas: if there are any T traumas in the partners' histories (i.e. earthquakes, attacks, accidents, miscarriage, etc.), it is required to process these events first.
- Target memories linked to the critical nucleus related to sexuality, i.e. to the deepest meaning connected to it, which can be traced back in both partners' attachment histories.
- Repetitive negative beliefs that come from each partner's primary attachment relationship (for instance, 'I am not that important', 'I do not deserve love').
- Current relational situations associated with the partner's particular behaviour that activate the negative schemes on the self, i.e. negative beliefs acquired on the self during infancy and triggered during the conflicts with the partner.
- Target memories directly connected to the sexual issue: first experiences, failures, traumas.

Phase 2: Preparation

Psychoeducation and explanation of the method

The couple must understand what is happening and what treatment is about. This psychoeducation work must include connecting the reported symptoms and problems on one side and the past and present experiences on the other. More importantly, in this phase, the couple must become more aware of their own functioning dynamics. Hence, the partners must be urged to explore and experiment sexuality since they often do not have appropriate knowledge of it, and it is experienced with embarrassment and, sometimes, even fear. The psychoeducation work must necessarily take into account the clients' age, which is a determining factor for the biological component of our sexuality since this consistently modifies the intensity and quality of the sexual reaction.

Many couples searching for help due to the wife's lacking reactivity or to rarer sexual intercourses simply suffer from their ignorance on sexual matters. Quite often, the partners do not know where the clitoris is located, or they cannot recognise its role as a transmitter of erotic pleasure. They get ready for coitus as soon as the husband has an erection, and the man ejaculates without considering how his partner is feeling in the sequence of her sexual reaction. These couples wonder, in good faith, why the woman cannot get a climax. Both partners contribute to this limited and inefficient sexual interaction. In fact, the woman does not ask for the stimulation she wants since she is not aware of her own needs and also because she is afraid that her husband can reject and abandon her if she admits she has some needs, which she herself could consider anomalous or selfish (Kaplan, 1974).

During therapy, the partners are encouraged to mutually communicate where and how they like to be caressed and what type of stimulation they want to try together. During therapy, the couple can explore the potential pleasure that lies in the possibility to vary the sexual experience depending on each partner's needs. The partners learn to enact alternated stimulation schemes on different occasions. The man must not 'hold back' every time; every now and then, he can reach climax quickly and then help his partner reach climax in turn later. The next time, the couple can dedicate time to slower foreplay to give the woman the possibility to experience her utmost pleasure. Misinformation exercises pressures on both husband and wife.

The therapist explains the EMDR method to the couple and provides the instructions on the procedure and on the modalities, which will be adopted, focusing on the couple's resources, strengthening self-observation and installing specific resources on the present stressors. To conclude, the therapist explains that some sessions will be for the couple, while others will entail work on the single partner. The therapist will assess whether the other partner's presence is required during reprocessing.

Identification of the resources

It is paramount to guarantee stabilisation of both partners and of the couple as a whole. Given that the relational work can activate the negative cognitions and the expression of the dissociated parts, some preparatory, preliminary individual sessions may be more effective before the partners' joint sessions. By enhancing the integrative capacity, the relational work becomes more constructive.

The therapeutic contract

Starting from the partners' individual request, the therapist must help them make their individual requests converge into a couple's request. It is paramount to find shared goals, whether the partners are staying together or splitting. The contract – i.e. cultivating motivation and the will to work towards change – is a very delicate step in therapy. Hence, the therapist must be aware that clients with dissociated parts may be ambivalent as for their will to change.

For some clients, a dissociated part can have a strong investment on the symptom and enough influence on the system of the self. Therefore, special techniques must be used to talk with the dissociated part to cultivate availability to heal and to change (for instance, the dissociative table technique, Fraser, 2003). The assessment defines the goals for the partners individually in addition to those for the couple. The therapist proposes a treatment plan for each partner and a relational plan for both. Later, they will have to negotiate 'who, what and when' regarding the therapeutic intervention. The partner starting the processing must be identified in a shared decision. If EMDR is conducted with one partner and the other is absent, the therapist will have to discuss the possibility for the excluded partner to contact the therapist and to be equally involved in therapy.

The work with the parts

During the work with the couple and in individual therapy as well, some sessions might have to be dedicated to identifying and integrating some dissociated parts of the self that can interfere with the attainment of the therapeutic goals agreed by the couple. These are parts of the personality that function according to often-childish modalities and strategies and that defend the individual without any benefit for the couple. These dissociative parts are activated within the couple relationship since the beginning; however, they are mainly expressed when the attachment relationship with the partner becomes more concrete and stable and when the initial phase of passion and falling in love leaves room to a routine couple relationship.

Those characteristics and traits of the other's personality that give the idea of an initial positive complementarity and that write the first chapters of the love story are soon replaced by an opposite perception, and they start the dysfunctional pathological dynamic that holds the couple under siege. What have the parts learnt? How does the couple work? What are the secondary advantages of the symptom? Working specifically on the symptom would mean strengthening the defensive and self-protective dissociated part in the other.

Quite often, the sexual dysfunction has the function to protect a part of the self, and this protects the client – in a dysfunctional way – from the risk to experience something that has been seen as dangerous before. The therapist must investigate what relational problems have had an impact on the sexual ones. Is the event causing the recent dysfunction? Is it part of the person's dysfunctionality? If the issue originated from an event in adulthood, it is easier. The dissociated parts often originate from reiterated traumas too.

When there is a conflict, there is often a high dissociative level. Being aware of the dissociated parts' dynamics can provide meaning to some puzzling behaviours and explain that a good therapy needs the whole system to collaborate. Since affect tolerance is strengthened, the partners can better use the joint relational therapy to learn how to talk, negotiate conflicts and stay tuned in front of the mutual individuality.

Phase 3: Assessment

Once identified the target events in the history of the couple and the sexual issue, the standard EMDR protocol phases follow in the order of priority defined earlier. It is then required to start from the target memories related to the partners' past history and to identify the present triggers in the current relationship, connected to the sexual dysfunction, by processing the past trigger memories and installing new positive scenarios connected to the current triggers. It is often useful to process the negative memories linked to the sexual dysfunction (first time, worst time, last time); this reduces performance anxiety and the fear to experience a moment of intimacy again.

Phases 4, 5 and 6: Desensitisation and reprocessing of the target event

During these phases, we have the peak moment in the processing of the event. The client moves progressively and alternatively from the past to the present, re-associating and reconnecting the events and information required to complete the filing of the event in an adaptive and functional way.

Phase 7: Closing

The actions listed next are part of the closing phase, which is dedicated to the partner who worked, the partner who assisted and the couple per *se*.

- Allow debriefing with the partner who worked, thus identifying all incomplete works and explaining that the internal processing could go on during the week (memories, dreams, etc.), and ask to take a note of all the emerging related material.
- Provide closing instructions and reflections to the passive partner, which do not include assessments or opinions, but only the expression of the moods and emotions felt during the session.
- Invite to share mutual appreciation, thus reinforcing one quality in the partner, which was appreciated during the session.
- Provide instructions to the couple on the time to elapse between two sessions and recommend avoiding discussions about the EMDR session in order not to interfere with the ongoing processing.

Phase 8: Revaluation

In this phase, a check is performed with both partners to assess whether it is required to have other EMDR sessions with the first partner before moving on to the second.

If possible, the therapist should keep some balance in the therapy and limit all EMDR processing shifts to two or three sessions per partner. Shifts can alternate several times along the couple's treatment.

7.4   The application of EMDR in couple's therapy

Introduction

The clinical case following hereto was selected because it represents the use of the EMDR protocol clearly in a case of vaginismus or sexless marriage. Therapy tackles the psychogenic aetiology of the disorder by focusing on its relational aspects, and at the same time, it offers both bodywork in collaboration with the gynaecologist and work on the couple's dynamics.

Phase 1: Individual and couple history taking

As given in Phase 1 in the EMDR protocol, information was collected on the couple's life history, Gaia and Marco, by focusing specifically on the two partners' attachment histories and on their relational and sexual dynamics. The goal in this phase is to gain the information required to conceptualise the case.

Referral

The couple was sent to therapy by the gynaecologist whom Gaia visited because she and her husband wanted to have a child. However, the doctor could not visit her. Gaia told the doctor that she had always avoided gynaecological visits and that she had never been able to have a full intercourse with her husband. The now commonly accepted multifactorial character of the sexual disorder, however, originated the need to approach the sexological client in an integrated way.

The therapy of sexual dysfunctions should take place constantly in a triadic relationship (doctor-psychologist-client), considering all the specific peculiarities implied in this situation (Bavestrello and Piccini, 1991). Consistent with the trend in contemporary science to process complex models instead of the reductive ones as in classical science, it is then desirable that the gynaecologist and the psychotherapist assume the psychosomatic nature of the sexual disorder and its multifactorial character, hence.

During the phone call, Gaia formulates her cry for help and presents a problematic situation in the sexual sphere of the relationship, 'I have a sexual problem'. Based on the first information collected on the phone, we decide to convene the couple.

Current problem (including duration and seriousness of the problem; Why treatment now?)

The couple comes to the first session. They have been married for three months after five years of engagement. They have never had other relationships. Gaia is 37 years old, but she looks much younger. She is a nursery schoolteacher, and she says she is happy with her work. Marco is 39. He also looks younger. He seems happy with his IT job in a bank, and he is available to talk about their situation. The problem that brought them to ask for help is their unconsummated marriage. During engagement, their sexual activity was scarce, with no attempts to coitus. After marriage, they have tried, but her great fear for pain emerged, accompanied by his fear to hurt her.

The explicit reason for the therapy request is her need to undergo a gynaecological examination and their great desire to have a baby. Gaia's drawing of her genitals shows great lack of anatomical knowledge: the vulva is sketched in a summary way, with no details (*Figure 7.1*). The diagnosis is 'primary vaginismus'; however, considering the husband, too, the most correct definition is 'sexless marriage'.

After the diagnostic interviews, Gaia undergoes couple psychotherapy to find new functioning schemes, apart from that including the doctor and sick Gaia; in fact, she pays her being 'sick' with suffering. However, she is also very powerful. She imposes herself the prohibition to try coitus until therapy is completed, to avoid additional frustrations and feelings of failure. The initial sessions aim at defining a cooperative alliance with the couple and at verbalising their emotional experiences, to identify the common goal and identify the attachment needs and meet them mutually inside the relationship. Probably, the request to move focus from sexuality to the couple allowed them to escape the prison of the symptom and extend their perspective.

After the symptomatic phase, the couple's conflict emerges more and more clearly. They are progressively recovering the possibility to talk openly about their needs and dissatisfactions that the symptomatic behaviour had always silenced and covered.

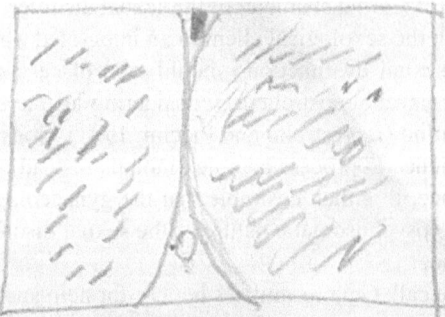

Figure 7.1 The first drawing of Gaia's genitals features dashed lines around the clitoral and vaginal area. The vagina is depicted as a black circle. There is a noticeable lack of understanding of its anatomy.

Family history and attachment relationships

Gaia describes her personal history as problematic, with some difficulties to separate from her family of origin, many parental conflicts and her father being absent, uninterested and violent. Marco appears passive, shy in his first experience with women, almost scared by the idea to harm his wife, however, a saviour for 'sick' Gaia; Marco lost his mother when he was very young, and he grew up with a cold, absent father. Emotional neglect, the fact of having only one reference parent and terror characterise the couple's childhood and seem to be common to both.

Negative childhood experiences (ACE) that occurred in the first years and in their evolution have probably led to the disorganisation of attachment and other internal motivational systems (IMS) in both. As regards the couple, the IMSs regulating their interactions appear almost fully or partially subverted. The attachment system should be aimed at asking for care, protection and comfort, and the caring system should provide them. The competitive system concerns competition targeted to define the social rank, while the cooperative system pursues the joint attainment of a shared goal. The sexual system tends to form and maintain the sexual couple.

Gaia seems to dominate in the couple through her hegemonic symptom. She seems to move within the competitive system, while asking for help and care. Marco, fully plunged into a dramatic triangle, appears like his wife's 'saviour' from her sickness; he does not insist on having sexual intercourse, so he does not become a 'perpetrator', and he ends up becoming the 'victim' of a sexless marriage.

Then their desire to have a child activates the attachment/caretaking system, and the couple focuses on the sexual issue that have always neglected or denied. The cooperative system is activated between the two individuals in the couple and the therapy team. Gaia's family history is complex and revolves around a never completed separation. Her attempts to 'leave' her affect and practical dependence on her family take place through several behaviours that reduce Gaia's margins of autonomy, trust and credibility. Marco enters Gaia's life with the goal to 'save her'. He is a smart and good man, not that handsome and not that self-confident. He forgets his uncertainties thanks to Gaia's 'sickness. Marco is interested in her as a sick, needy person. Gaia accepts Marco's protection, however, not his passivity. Gaia talks about the continuous conflicts between her parents, and she feels strong resentment against her father. She has not seen him for four years, and she has always accused him to be violent and never interested in their family. Instead, Gaia has always had a strong relationship with her mother, and she has even shared her bedroom with her for many years. Gaia has grown up with female reference figures (mother and elder sister) because her father was often away for work. This fact is very important because she believes she has taken up all their criticism against men.

In Marco's family history, a 'T' trauma occurs when he is 7 years old: his mother had cancer, and she died six months after the diagnosis. The family reacts to mourning by establishing the reign of silence. Given the family context of his evolution,

Marco has come to believe that it is more convenient for him not to talk about his problems and suffering with others. It is better to keep everything for himself, and this is aimed mostly at not originating additional concerns for his father, who had already been disturbed by his own personal events.

Sexological assessment

The assessment shows a difficulty in communicating their own needs and sexual preferences. In their answers to the different items, both partners report that their families of origin had a negative view of the body, of sexual expression and of intimacy. Marco's father has never been a good interlocutor for such issues, and he appeared quite embarrassed when talking about these topics. His mother's early death made it impossible for Marco to confront a woman figure on these topics. Gaia's mother – who is extremely religious – provided her with a very rigid and closed sexual education. She did not even inform her daughter on menstruations, sexual intercourses and contraception. During puberty, Gaia never allowed herself to experience masturbation since she considered the exploration of her body as possibly negative and 'dirty'.

Marco never forced penetration, for fear of harming his wife, traumatising her and, hence, worsening the situation. Of course, he is not aware of the strong collusion that has originated between them in this way. Gaia knows that vaginismus is her problem, and she clearly feels the muscle contraction in her pelvic area when Marco attempts penetration. She cannot tolerate pain of any kind; hence, she is frightened just by thinking about feeling pain.

All penetration attempts have failed because Gaia felt a strong pain whenever he simply approached her, and Marco never wanted to force her. It has also been impossible for him to introduce a finger into her vagina. Marco spontaneously says that he now understands he used Gaia's refusal as an excuse to hide his fears related to sexuality; however, he has never suffered from erectile dysfunctions or similar sexual dysfunctions. During all these years, Marco has never thought about trying to have sex with another woman, and he acknowledges that Gaia is his first woman and that he has been blocked for years since he did not know how to win over his shyness.

Risk and/or maintenance factors

We analyse the meaning and function of the symptom inside the psychic economy at the individual, couple and family levels and in the transition of the vital cycle, which entails a reorganisation in the couple. Both partners place themselves in the phase, which literature (Malagoli Togliatti and Cotugno, 1996) defines as the phase when the couple is formed. These two young adults have been married for three months, and for sure, they are experiencing the phase of reorganising their interpersonal relationships and of 'directing their affect and organisation investments into the new couple-family'.

The disorders related to the neurotic area that fall in the 'category' of the disorders a young couple suffers from during the consolidation phase and that show up more evidently in this phase are those typical of sexual dysfunctions. The difficulties this couple is facing are connected to the meaning they have given to their marriage, which is used as an attempt to separate from their families of origin. There is an internal contradiction between a state of mind where they have found some sort of balance and a persistent dissatisfaction.

Apart from Gaia's stated difficulties, the partner – who is little autonomous from an emotional point of view, sexually undemanding and subdued – strongly colluded with the symptom of vaginismus for many years. Both are asked what is more serious for them: Gaia's vaginismus or Marco's inability to act in this situation to eliminate Gaia's issue, which is obliging them to pay a lot in terms of role rigidity. Gaia shows a great deal of scepticisms, not towards psychotherapy but in regards to her ability to solve the problem. She feels discouraged, and she believes she is not like other women. She really loves her husband, but she thinks he would have been able to help her if he had been more experienced.

Identification of the target memories and of the therapeutic plan

During the history taking phase, our focus on the memories connected to Gaia's experience of violence inside the family during childhood becomes more and more crucial. Significant target memories emerge linked to father's violence against her mother, elder sister and herself and to Gaia's perceived 'lack of control'. That 'control' is now exercised on her body through the distance she wants to keep from her husband. Gaia has never been able to reprocess the anger she felt for her distant and strongly hated father. Hence, it is fundamental to identify the future target memories we will have to work on. Gaia understands that her lacking trust towards her father has been automatically extended to all men.

In Marco's childhood, the most significant target memories are linked to his mother's disease (cancer) and the big T trauma of grief when he was 7 years old. Another target event connected to the negative cognition 'I am not good enough' is the memory dating back to age 8: he had obtained a very good mark at school, but his father had remained indifferent. Here is Marco's description of his father: 'I have grown up without ever being appreciated by my father. He has never encouraged me. Never a sign of his love'.

The most significant traumatic memories in Marco's family history are his mother's early death when he was a child, the difficulties to identify with his father – whom he describes as cold and absent – and the lacking family models from which he could differentiate. He acknowledges the impact these events have had on his life, and this helps Marco understand better his sense of inadequacy and his relational difficulties to women.

In short:

- Identification of the trigger event (recent gynaecological check-up linked to their desire to have a baby).
- T traumas:

  Gaia: witnessed violence (her father's violence against her mother and elder sister); an episode when her father pushed her against the wardrobe, causing her a mild concussion (age 6); the memory of a sexual abuse by her father (age 7) emerged only later.
  Marco: blocked grief for his mother's death (age 7).

- Target memories linked to the critical nucleus related to sexuality, i.e. to its deepest meaning and which can be found in both partners' attachment history:

  Gaia: her first menstruations and her fear when she saw the blood; mother did not tell her about the menstrual cycle (age 12); mother discovered that Gaia had kissed a boy and she told her that she was 'easy' (age 15).
  Marco: a memory of his father changing the TV channel when an explicit sexual scene was shown in the movie (age 15).

- Repetitive negative beliefs coming from each partner's primary attachment relationship: 'I have no control'. Episode: father suddenly left home after a violent discussion (age 10). Episode: mother cried desperately after father had beaten her (age 8).

  Marco: 'I am not good enough'. Episode: father remained indifferent in front of a very good mark from school (age 8). 'I do not trust my body . . . I am weak', a somatic weakness construction. This construction seems to be supported by a perception: both uncertainty/vulnerability (probably affected by earlier experiences of both physical and psychological traumatic wounds) and scarce reactive readiness, i.e. activation (affected by his excessive weight) of the physical resources required for sexual intercourses.

- Current relational situations (*triggers*) associated with a special behaviour of the partner that activate negative patterns on the self, i.e. negative beliefs gained of their own self during childhood and triggered during the conflicts with the partner:

  Gaia: Marco's silence activates the negative belief 'I do not deserve attention'.
  Marco: Gaia's distracted expression activates the belief 'I am not important'.

- Target memories directly connected to the sexual issue: first experiences, failures, traumas.

  Gaia: memory of when she found her father watching a porn movie one evening (age 10), first attempt of a complete intercourse when she felt a very strong pain and she burst into tears (age 20), her mother's storytelling on the fact that her father was 'fixated' with sex (age 30).

Marco: joking at by his peers (age 14); his schoolmate refuses to kiss him (age 15); first sexual experience failed with a girl at university (age 25); target memories of his friends who started joking at him after discovering he had never had sex (age 28); feeling of powerlessness during his first sexual approach (age 39).

The couple's functioning

According to the results of Sternberg's test, both partners state that they are equally 'committed' to the couple relationship, and the 'commitment' variable score is above average. The 'intimacy' variable is slightly below average. The test shows that both share interests and values. They feel mutual total trust and tend to take care of the other. The items connected to an open communication of their emotions show some gaps.

As regards 'passion', the scores are significantly below average for both. A difficulty emerges that is connected not only to physical attraction but to sexual desire too. In addition, a strong idealisation emerges. In fact, there are some very high scores in Gaia's 'ideal' triangle, showing a desire for great closeness, an extreme search for full intimacy and total sharing.

Couple affect regulation strategies

When affect regulation does not develop correctly, the individual must defend from specific experiences that cause specific emotions. This prevents the integration between the event and the related emotion; the emotions linked to the event thus become dysregulated and lead to dissociative or impulsive reactions, or they are removed (Hughes, 2012).

Some clients' narrations often show inconsistent emotions emerging as for the reported event. To frame their affect regulation strategies, both partners are asked to reflect on some significant episodes that have triggered intense dysregulated emotions.

'What behaviours, words and expressions typical of your partner activate dysregulated responses? Are there any behaviours, words or facial expressions that make you feel humiliated, inferior, subdued? What emotions do you feel in these situations? How do you feel after these reactions?'

Gaia feels a strong sensation of control loss during their sexual approaches. When Marco approaches her and touches on her more intensely, she feels a strong sense of powerlessness and reacts by regaining immediate control of the situation.

'Do you experience such control loss with frustration and shame or with humiliation? Can you think about what child experience triggered the same feelings in you?'

Gaia is moved and she talks about some memories of her father's violence. She acknowledges that talking about them is enough to make her feel anguished.

As concerns Marco, the detached expression on his wife's face when she briskly pushes him away during the sexual approach makes him feel 'inferior'. The float-back on the negative cognition ('I am disappointing') and on the associated sensation shows significant memories connected to his attachment history. Marco also recognises his trend to caring as a tool to meet his need for closeness.

Gaia and Marco are asked to bring a list of relational triggers in the following session, which are associated with the partner's disturbing behaviour. For each trigger, the negative beliefs gained of their own self during childhood and activated during the conflicts with the partner are identified. Marco complains about the fact that Gaia never listens to him. He is then asked how this makes him feel, and Marco admits that in those moments, he feels like he is not worth anything at all. He is not important. Marco is asked to observe what he notes in his body when he thinks about the words 'I am not important' and if there is an image that accompanies the perceived physical sensation. Marco remembers when he was little and his father was always busy. He used to tell him what had happened at school, but his father was always distracted.

Gaia is asked if she knows that Marco perceives he is unworthy when she does not listen to him. As a response, Gaia tenderly moves her hand towards her husband. Partners do not always become aware that the emotions they experience come from their past (Attili, 2011). During the following sessions, we try to identify and remove the obstacles in the spouses' communication to facilitate higher affect tuning.

Identification of individual and couple resources

Learning to calm down and to calm their own emotional states is an important relational skill. To learn it, it is paramount to work first on their own activating triggers. It is important to work with both partners and identify the moments when the partner was caring and empathic (Fosha, 2016) and the positive relational experiences, i.e. when the partner was supportive and comforting. Both can identify the moments when they worked well as a couple to restore the positive perception of their relationship, even only partially. This enhances the alliance inside the couple and fosters stabilisation and preparation to process both the individual and the couple's wounds.

Phase 2: Preparation

This phase is devoted to explaining EMDR to both partners since it was paramount that they could understand the treatment in order to strengthen their personal and couple motivations. During this psychoeducational work, we highlighted and explained the connection between symptoms and reported issues and between past and present experiences. To conclude, we underlined the importance to focus on the identification and strengthening of both individual and couple resources.

Resource identification (RDI)

Before processing target memories with EMDR, Gaia and Marco had five sessions to identify and install resources through the RDI protocol to foster the initial stabilisation of the current situation by acquiring better affect regulation and coping skills (Korn and Leeds, 2002; Leeds and Shapiro, 2000). The first resource to be installed was the 'safe place'. Then the resources were identified to address their current difficulties, and both partners were asked to identify their positive personal qualities that would be helpful. Marco acknowledged his need to be more assertive and to improve his relational skills. During the RDI sessions, he was asked to focus on his specific positive autobiographical memories where he felt he could access the desired qualities and resources. By using the RDI protocol, the following resources were installed and strengthened: the perception of a skilled, adequate adult state and the feelings and affects associated with it. The resource was identified in the memory of his election to class representative and of his ability to convince the professors to bring the class on a trip abroad.

Gaia would like to rely more on others, and during the sessions, she identified a memory to this purpose: she had started an internship with her dance mates and managed to let herself go fully into dancing.

EMDR sessions

Psychotherapy includes both couple's sessions and alternated individual sessions with Gaia and with Marco, in which EMDR is used to process the traumatic events.

Working with parts

In couple's work, therapy differentiates if a partner shows an important history, or his/her history memories are quite complete.

During Marco's individual sessions, the standard EMDR protocol was used, while with Gaia – as we will describe here later – it was essential to work with the parts. Gaia was helped to trace back and describe an internal safe place where her parts could feel safe and discuss and be accessible, following Fraser's dissociative table technique (1991) as a model. By talking to the therapist and through a more and more aware space-time orientation, Gaia was able to create an internal safe place where she could acknowledge all her parts, their roles, pain, resources and goals. The development of awareness, co-conscience and compassion between the different parts of the self was paramount.

During the first individual sessions with Gaia, her excessive alertness towards affect and sexual closeness led us to assume a dissociative amnesia since the very beginning, in which the 'emotional part' (EP) fixated on the trauma and on the defensive systems was separated from the 'apparently normal part' (ANP) that allowed her to go on with her daily life. Gaia's excessive alertness prevented accessing the memories connected to the traumatic experience. The dissociative response represents an automatic response that – in time – turns into a model response to emotions and situations that often lead the person to unprocessed painful events. Gaia had immediately shown the 'control part' with a defensive protective function against the intense emotions associated with painful traumatic memories. It was believed that creating an alliance with the 'control part' would allow Gaia to experience the therapist as a less dangerous figure and to preserve the therapeutic alliance that was gradually being formed.

We started by processing the target memories of her attachment history to help Gaia activate the initial processing and connections between the 'mental states' in a field where she feels safer, leading her carefully to access a very traumatic past later.

Following the RDI sessions and the part work, we selected the painful memories identified both during the attachment history taking phase and during the work with the same parts. We applied the standard EMDR protocol to each target event, from Phase 3 to 8 (Shapiro, 2001). The attachment history showed the absence of safety in the significant relationships and the lacking tuning with the caregiver, which can be associated with a disorganised attachment.

After some sessions when we worked on the 'shame' part, Gaia was back to therapy and reported she had had several nightmares and she was feeling very confused and anguished. We gave her a blank sheet of paper, and we asked her to make a drawing to represent the experience she was having in that moment. Gaia drew this drawing very quickly (*Figure 7.2*) and burst into tears, confessing that the memory of her father's abuse when she was 7 had emerged. Hence, drawing had

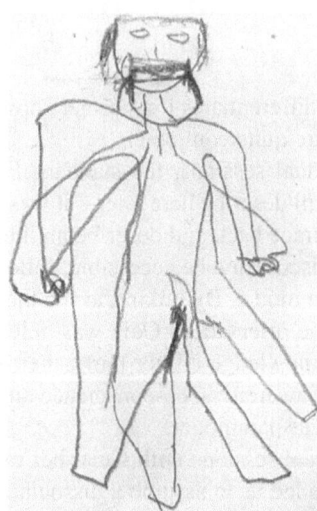

Figure 7.2 Gaia draws two human figures: her father standing behind her, leaning on her genital area. In the drawing, the father's eyes are visible, while Gaia's face is blank, without eyes, nose or mouth. There is a dark shading in the genital area. Neither her father's feet nor her own are depicted in the drawing.

been very helpful for the client, as it had allowed her to express and share the chaos and confusion in her internal world.

In this case, Gaia's therapeutic path is somehow divided into two distinct moments: the first is when the traumatic event was fully estranged from con-science; the second is when a flashback neatly showed the image of an abuse that had been fully removed. By restarting the work with the parts, the client had a spontaneous abreaction, and it was important to contain it, to introduce the elements for reality orientation, by strengthening this state and encouraging the introduction of another stronger part that could help the weaker one tackle the traumatic elements.

Since the moment when the abuse memories emerged, processing the worst images associated with that event has allowed her to reprocess the memories associated with the childhood trauma and to transform the negative cognitions on lacking safety into new positive cognitions on her ability to provide herself with protection and calmness.

Therapy continued with couple's meetings to help the client emotionally share her work and to differentiate her husband from her father figure. This allowed her to start perceiving her husband's passion without fear, which used to activate dis-sociative aspects in her.

The integrated approach to vaginismus

Some check-ups are planned with the gynaecologist in the team that will have to be performed during this phase of therapy. In fact, it will be required to lead Gaia through an appropriate preparation course to get to know her body. Three moments are planned: the first meeting will allow us to check only that her external genitals are normal and that no anatomical anomalies are present (actually, they are quite rare, but they are often present as ghosts in the experience of women with vaginis-mus). During the second check-up, Gaia will be encouraged to introduce her finger into her vagina and to allow the doctor to do the same thereafter. During the third check-up, a full gynaecological visit will be performed with the introduction of the *speculum* and the execution of a smear test.

The collaboration with the gynaecologist is precious because the client gener-ally needs that a doctor concretely checks the attained results and the real possibil-ity to 'open' the vagina. In this phase of the therapy, it is paramount to strengthen the resources and increase body awareness through the following exercises:

- 'Four elements' exercise for stress management (Elan Shapiro).
- Respiratory training, relaxation exercises, body awareness and exercises to change the dysfunctional respiratory patterns.
- Exercises to increase body awareness in general and the awareness of the pelvic area specifically.

As expected, the first phase of therapy showed Gaia's phobic structures and her husband's difficulties to contain emotions. Hence, we continued with the individual therapy, and Gaia gradually learnt to watch and touch her genitals in front of a mirror with the help of Kegel exercises. The first gynaecological check-up was experienced with much anxiety and apprehension; however, it was very useful because Gaia felt reassured about her anatomically normal genitals.

Treatment continued quite well, and Gaia committed a lot to perform the assigned tasks. However, every session showed an intense experience of inadequacy that brought her to be very pessimistic and not able to valorise the results she had attained. It was fundamental to perform continuous emotional strengthening work and to provide explanations on the need to learn to tolerate pain. This phase of treatment aimed to reduce/eliminate pain and to reformulate the relationship with sexuality by the following:

• Processing some traumatic events connected to the perceived pain.
• Applying Mark Grant's EMDR protocol for pain (2023).
• Experiential part with the pelvic rehabilitator.

By applying the EMDR protocol for pain, Gaia started to increase her abilities to control and manage actual pain. In this phase of individual psychotherapy sessions, it was fundamental to use *drawings* as a therapeutic response to allow representing her vagina and the moment of penetration. The drawing became the target to be processed with the EMDR protocol. The use of drawings allowed Gaia to represent her phobia and helped her identify specific disturbing aspects connected to her perception of genitals.

Gaia drew *Figure 7.3* during a session when she was trying to express how one of her parts had been able to have control over her body by creating a cloud enveloping it and a 'wall' (fence) to defend her further from additional external dangers (arrows and little men). Moreover, during some sessions, starting from the disturbance caused by the drawing, it was possible to complete a float-back and trace back to significant trigger memories, thus reprocessing them with the EMDR protocol.

The progression of these drawings (*Figure 7.4, 7.5* and *7.6*) shows the changes that prepared Gaia for the following steps.

When Gaia learnt to introduce one finger into her vagina, we decided to pass on to the second gynaecological examination. It was a very important moment for her because the gynaecologist gave her more strength by informing her positively on the results she had attained. As agreed, the examination was partial; hence, it took place without introducing the speculum (which was postponed to a later moment). After Gaia acquired the mental image of the penis in the vagina, we decided to involve the husband in the therapy again.

Marco actively participated in the sessions. He committed to performing the assigned tasks at home. He was very precise in writing down and reporting moods and emotions, and he accepted to show more firmness towards his wife.

After some attempts, Marco was stuck and entered in contact with his anxiety and with a feeling of inadequacy, while Gaia did not take up all the responsibilities for what was happening. Instead, she assigned a part of what had happened during

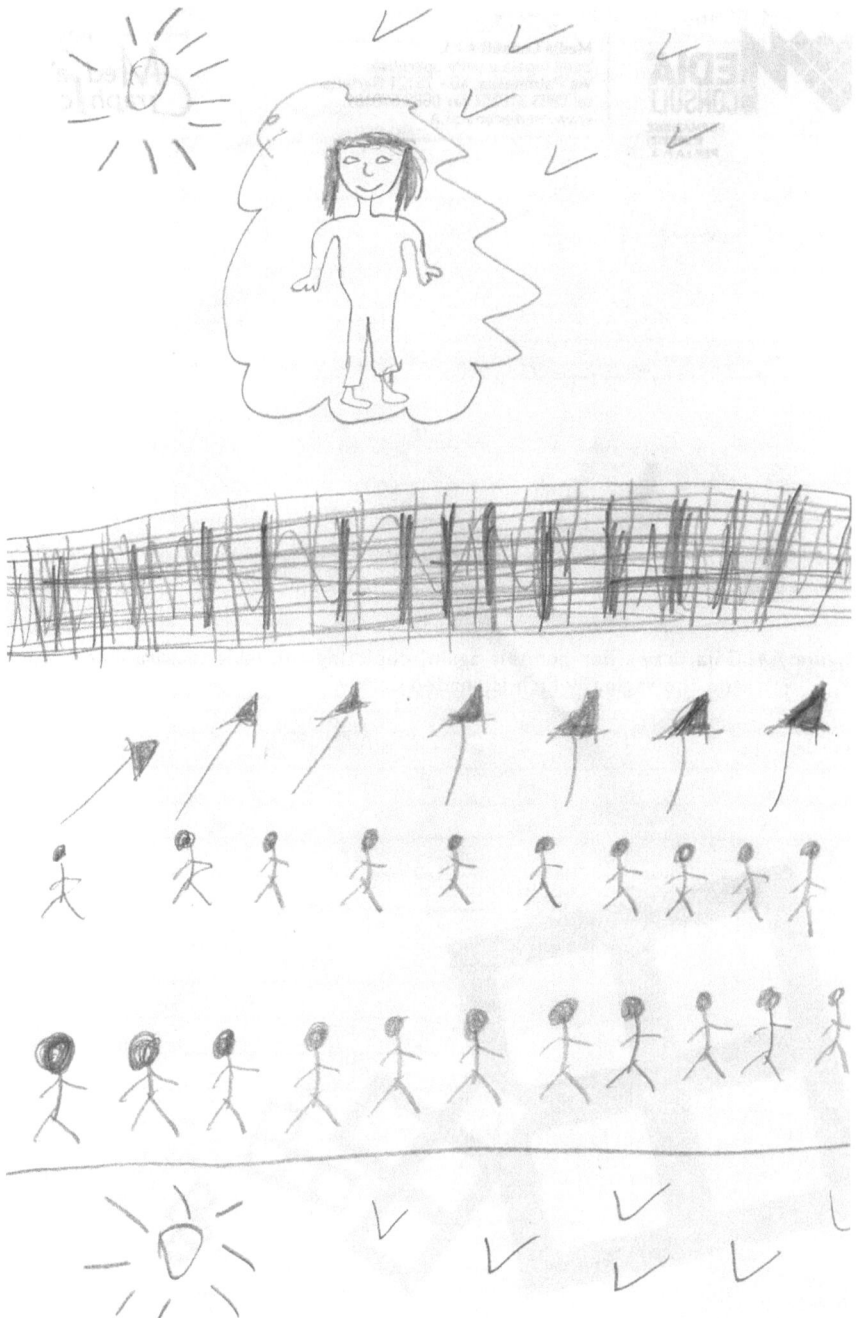

Figure 7.3 At the top of the drawing, Gaia is inside a cloud. Next to her in the sky are swallows and the sun. In the middle section, there is a fence that protects her from external dangers (the arrows and the stick figures) depicted in the lower part of the drawing. At the bottom of the page, separated from the middle section, the sun and swallows are shown again.

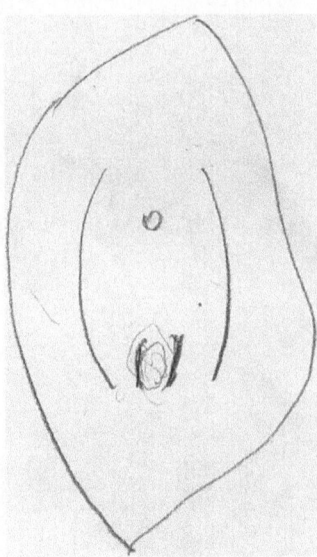

Figure 7.4 Gaia draws her genitals again, depicting the labia majora, the clitoris and the vagina, which is shaded darkly.

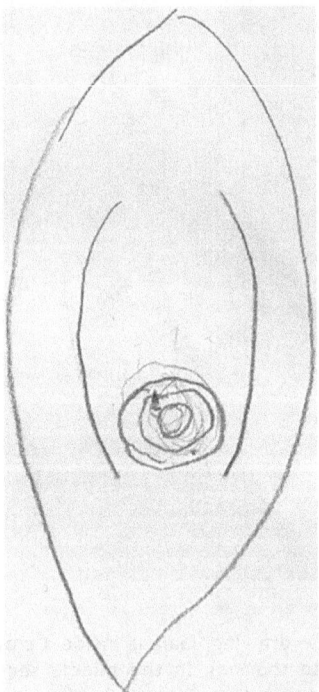

Figure 7.5 Gaia draws her genitals, depicting the labia majora. The clitoris is absent, but the vagina is prominently marked, with three overlapping circles.

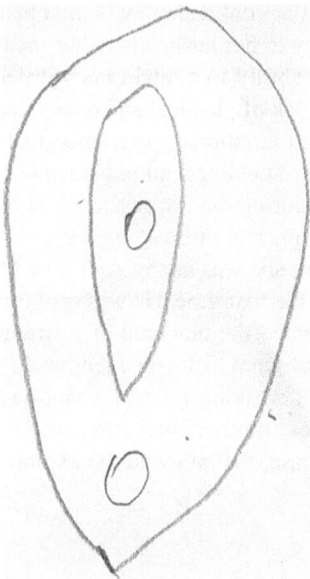

Figure 7.6 Gaia draws her genitals for the last time, depicting the labia majora, the clitoris and the vagina. The lines in the drawing are consistent across all areas, with no intense shading.

the sexual intercourse to her husband. Gaia led Marco to introduce a finger into her vagina without her feeling any pain but only some tolerable discomfort. Additional sessions were required to strengthen these results and to reflect together on the dynamic of their relationship.

Gaia became more aware of the contradiction between holding a dominant position on her husband and, at the same time, pretending more safety and authoritativeness on his side. We worked a lot on both partners finding their autonomous spaces, with the goal to attain a higher level of differentiation. At this point, the third gynaecological check-up was performed with the introduction of the speculum without any problems. The smear test was completed without any difficulties, and the proposal to try penetration was welcomed. After a couple of attempts, it was successful without Gaia experiencing any much-feared pain. Gaia noticed she had become more self-confident, and she felt like a 'real woman'.

The couple told us that the intercourse anxiety had gradually left room to their desire to be close, which they had never experienced before.

Discussion

The approach to the person as a whole by availing of different professional figures allowed us to provide an extremely effective clinical response. Integrated therapy allowed Gaia to activate and recognise calmness and to become more aware of her body. Gaia acquired more confidence by being open to more exploration, thus assigning less responsibility to her husband for her 'healing'. Marco showed firmness and strengthened his ability to contain his wife emotionally. Gaia was then calm enough to tackle the risk of physical and psychological pain.

EMDR allowed a shared emotional experience that brought to an increase in tuning, hence, a deeper understanding, compassion and contact ability. The partners seemed to be quite at ease during the last session, and both reported improvements still under way. Gaia said they had made some restructuring works, and even if her father-in-law opposed them, she was happy with how Marco had supported her: 'I felt I was not alone . . . for the first time. He was supporting me and not his father'.

Home restructuring seemed the outcome of a strengthened life project, and it represented the metaphor of what had happened inside the couple. Since they had 'restructured' their internal working models as individuals and as a couple and they had tuned their internal motivational systems, Gaia and Marco could share a common house, a 'safe base' that allowed the exploration of the outside and the projection into the future.

Revaluation

A follow-up was planned after three months from the last session to check how the couple had changed and evolved.

At the follow-up, the couple was very serene: Gaia felt she was living her femininity in full, and Marco felt safer in their relationship. The attained identification no longer activated those protective mechanisms that had been at the base of their union. New ways of being together were found because the old ones did not work anymore.

After one year, Gaia said she was pregnant and in her fourth month, and even though she was very afraid of the delivery, she felt safer, and she could live it fully as a woman. In addition, she saw that Marco was ready to be with her in this new phase of their growth.

Please note that the names chosen for the narration of the clinical cases are invented due to privacy reasons.

7.5 Clinical application of Sternberg's triangle

Clinical triangle's application

The triangle is used as a basic structure for later work. At first, it is used to check the level of commitment and to understand what the lacking aspects are in the love relationship. In the process of describing the triangle, the clinician must formulate five diagnostic questions, which can be asked directly or indirectly depending on the therapist's style.

1. The first question is if both partners want to experience all the three parts in the triangle. There are evident cases where one partner denies any involvement or shows no sexual interest in the other.

2. The second question is if each partner wants to experience each part in the triangle with the same intensity. The partners must be asked if they think they want the same level of intensity in the three areas or if they feel there are any discrepancies. The clinician should notice if one or more areas is/are given too much or too little relevance. When there are some discrepancies, the therapist must lead the couple towards a common agreement on the related levels.
3. The third question concerns what prevents the identification and expression of these three parts. Each partner should be able to identify and define the three parts and speak about each part openly and freely. Many couples can identify and define a component at intellectual level; however, the partners may not be correspondingly able to express it at emotional and behavioural level too. The therapist should ask the partners to think about what prevents them from expressing some specific feelings.
4. The fourth question is if each partner has a realistic perception of what love implies. Some partners think about love in a highly distorted and not very realistic way.
5. The fifth question is if both partners have a realistic perception of who they are and what they have been able to offer. When the couple speaks about the three areas, the partner's feedback and the way the couple interacts will provide information on the limitations.

Sternberg's triangular love scale – instructions

Blank spaces represent the person with whom you are having a relationship. Rate your agreement with each statement twice on a 1-to-9 scale, where 1 is not at all, 5 is moderate and 9 is extreme. Use the other scores in the scale to indicate intermediate levels of feelings.

The first score should represent how much the given statement is *characteristic* of your relationship. In other words, to what extent does a given statement reflect the way you feel in the relationship?

The second score should represent how much the given statement is *important* for your relationship. In other words, how much do you feel it is important that you feel that way, independent of how you truly feel?

Intimacy/Passion/Commitment Scheme

'Intimacy' questionnaire

1. I am actively supportive of . . . .'s well-being.
2. I have a warm relationship with . . . .
3. I am able to count on . . . . in times of need.
4. . . . . is able to count on me in times of need.
5. I am willing to share myself and my possessions with . . . .
6. I receive considerable emotional support from . . . .
7. I give considerable emotional support to . . . .

8. I communicate well with . . . .
9. I value . . . . greatly in my life.
10. I feel close to . . . .
11. I have a comfortable relationship with . . . .
12. I feel that I really understand . . . .
13. I feel that . . . . really understands me.
14. I feel that I can really trust . . . .
15. I share deeply personal information about myself with . . . .

'Passion' questionnaire

16. Just seeing . . . . excites me.
17. I find myself thinking about . . . . frequently during the day.
18. My relationship with . . . . is very romantic.
19. I find . . . . to be very personally attractive.
20. I idealise . . . .
21. I cannot imagine another person making me as happy as . . . .
    . . . . does.
22. I would rather be with . . . . than with anyone else.
23. There is nothing more important to me than my relationship with . . . .
24. I especially like physical contact with . . . .
25. There is something almost 'magical' about my relationship with . . . .
26. I adore . . . .
27. I cannot imagine life without . . . .
28. My relationship with . . . . is passionate.
29. When I see romantic movies and read romantic books, I think of . . . .
30. I fantasise about . . . .

'Commitment' questionnaire

31. I know that I care about . . . .
32. I am committed to maintaining my relationship with . . . .
33. Because of my commitment to . . . ., I would not let other
    people come between us.
34. I have confidence in the stability of my relationship with . . . .
35. I could not let anything get in the way of my commitment to . . . .
36. I expect my love for . . . . to last for the rest of my life.
37. I will always feel a strong responsibility for . . . .
38. I view my commitment to . . . . as a solid one.
39. I cannot imagine ending my relationship with . . . .

40. I am certain of my love for . . . .
41. I view my relationship with . . . . as permanent.
42. I view my relationship with . . . . as a good decision.
43. I feel a sense of responsibility toward . . . .
44. I plan to continue my relationship with . . . .
45. Even when . . . . is hard to deal with, I remain committed to our relationship.

Scoring

Items from 1 to 15 in the scale measure the 'intimacy' part, from 16 to 30 the 'passion' part and from 31 to 45 the 'decision/commitment' part.

To obtain the score for each part, add up the scores for each item and divide the result by 15. Thus, you will have an average for each item (outside the context of this book, the scale items are not grouped together by components, but they are given in erratic order).

The scale rules

Here is the information we have collected. It is given separately by *characteristic* and *importance*. Ideally, the level of each information being characteristic of the relationship should correspond generally to the level of the same being important for the same relationship. Of course, the more the important aspects are characteristics of a relationship, the larger the partners' satisfaction. Alternatively, the higher the gap between the items' characteristic and importance, the higher the potential discomfort and suffering.

Characteristics

Alt Text: The second table focuses on the extent to which each piece of information characterizes the importance of the relationship. It includes the three dimensions of the couple (intimacy, passion, and commitment) and the corresponding scores (high, low, and medium).

How characteristic of your relationship is each statement?

	Intimacy	Passion	Commitment
High	8.6	8.2	8.7
Medium	7.4	6.5	7.2
Low	6.2	4.9	5.7

Importance

Alt Text: The first table focuses on the extent to which each piece of information characterizes the relationship. It includes the three dimensions of the couple (intimacy, passion, and commitment) and the corresponding scores (high, low, and medium).

How important is each statement for your relationship?

	Intimacy	Passion	Commitment
High	9.0	8.0	8.8
Medium	8.2	6.8	7.6
Low	7.4	5.4	6.5

With reference to the individuals we tested, we have reported about 15% of high scores, 15% of low scores and about 70% of moderate scores.

7.6   Checklist for the couple's sexological assessment

With reference to the sexological assessment mentioned in Phase 1 of the treatment, here follows a checklist of the main investigation fields that the therapist will have to analyse during the clinical interview.

1. Definition of the problem.
2. Physical health (with possible deeper medical investigations if required, particularly in case of erection disorders).
3. Possible drug taking.
4. The family members' attitudes and education as regards sexuality: communication modalities, attitude towards nakedness at home, pre-marriage sexual activity, masturbation, homosexuality, etc.
5. Modalities to learn the main notions on sexuality and reproduction (changes occurring during puberty, during menstruations, nocturnal emissions) from the following: parents, teachers, peers, etc.
6. Religious beliefs as regards attitudes on sexuality (masturbation, petting, pre-marriage sex, abortion, contraception, etc.).
7. Beliefs related to specific aspects of sexuality: distinction between sexual roles in taking the sexual initiative (i.e. the man must always act first); the importance assigned to the penis size to please a woman; the (wrong) belief according to which a man must be able to keep his erection throughout sexual intercourse after he has attained it (otherwise, the man must have a problem, or the woman is not enough exciting for him); the belief that the climax must necessarily take place during the sexual intercourse or however following penetration; attitudes towards oral/anal practices, etc.; the (wrong) belief that simultaneous climax is the best and 'correct' way to attain sexual satisfaction.

8. Beliefs on the distinctions between 'male' and 'female' sexual roles. Possibly existing 'double standards'.

9. History of past sexual and/or affect experiences and of the related sexual satisfaction.

10. History of the current affect/sexual relationship and of the past and present sexual satisfaction with the current partner.

11. Modalities to attain climax: alone, with the partner, vaginal or clitoral orgasm.

12. Satisfaction as for the frequency and quality of their own orgasm. Comparison with the satisfaction about its frequency and quality in past sexual experiences, with other partners and with the current one. Possible dissatisfaction in case the sexual intercourse does not sometimes end with a climax (analysing reactions, whether the unattained climax is one's own or the partner's).

13. The need that orgasm is reached through penetration or accepting that it can be reached in other ways (or in a way by one partner and in a different way by another). The need to reach climax for the sexual intercourse to be considered satisfactory.

14. Importance to make the partner feel pleasure. Need to notice that you have been able to induce pleasure in the partner before feeling it.

15. Possible current masturbation practices (sexual activity without a partner) and satisfaction/dissatisfaction with them. Attitude on masturbation, even in adulthood if there is a sexual partner. Possible feelings of guilt related to past and present masturbation.

16. Satisfactory frequency of sexual intercourses with the partner.

17. Do the two partners have the same needs as regards the frequency of sexual intercourses?

18. Do one of the two partners sometimes accept sex even though he/she does not feel like it?

19. Does one of the partners sometimes pretend to feel pleasure even if he/she does not feel it in reality?

20. How does the partner inform that he/she does not want to have sex? What are the partner's reactions?

21. Do the partners generally talk about their own sexual sphere?

22. Are there any erotic fantasies? When? How often? Are they exciting? Do they cause discomfort? Does the person having them approve?

23. Are there any dreams with sexual content? How often?

24. What are the hygienic practices before and after sex?

25. Does their own nakedness cause discomfort? Why? When?

26. Does the partner's nakedness cause discomfort? Why? When?

27. What is the level of satisfaction related to one's own body? And to the partner's body?

28. Do the partners believe they are physically attractive for their own partner? And vice versa?

29. Are there any external obstacles (like lacking privacy or appropriate places) to a good outcome for the couple's sexual relationship?

30. Are sexual intercourses consummated particularly during some days or periods? Are there any days or periods when they are not consummated?
31. Any possible contraceptive methods used and their level of satisfaction.
32. Attitudes and beliefs about homosexuality.
33. Have you ever felt sexual attraction for a same-sex person? Was this a cause for worry?
34. Possible use of external means to attain sexual excitement: readings, magazines, videos, alcohol, drugs, partner swapping, group sex, etc. Does the partner share these practices?
35. Possible paraphilic sexual arousal (this area needs to be investigated with special care since it may not be stated spontaneously given the paraphilics' egosynthonicity).
36. Assessment of one's own sexual desire on a scale from 0 (totally absent) to 10 (extremely high desire). Estimate the partner's sexual desire on a scale from 0 (totally absent) to 10 (extremely high).
37. Assessment of the intensity of the orgasm on a scale from 0 (totally absent) to 10 (extremely high). Estimate the partner's intensity of orgasm on a scale from 0 (totally absent) to 10 (extremely high).
38. Assessment of their own sexual satisfaction on a scale from 0 (totally absent) to 10 (extremely high). Estimate the partner's sexual satisfaction on a scale from 0 (totally absent) to 10 (extremely high).

7.7   EMDR protocol for disorders with sexual pain – treatment

The connection between trauma and pain is more evident on a body level. The treatment of pain includes psychotherapeutic work on the meaning of the felt pain, a protocol on pain with the analysis of its components, regaining their own body sensations through self-recognition of tensions with the use of techniques to contract rigid muscles and the processing of traumatic events with EMDR.

In sexuality, both psychological and physical factors are strictly related. Conflicts and fear of sex and sexuality, often due to previous abuse, and relational problems are shown through the body language, through pain that prevents or limits the partner's access to their own body or prevents and blocks the perception of pleasure.

We know that trauma is an experience that – within a short time – contributes to psychic life with a strong increase in stimuli whose processing cannot be performed in the usual way.

If a critical event occurs within a situation of previous vulnerability, an alarm reaction sets off, with the following increased muscular tension, and there will be a cognitive distortion of the event. If the alarm is maintained, muscular tension increases, and hypertonia causes physical pain with an additional increase in muscular tension and, hence, in pain. Painful somatisations often include psychogenic muscular dystonia, i.e. a contraction of some muscular groups, which can cause structural alterations in the corresponding parts on the long run.

Sexual disorders due to genital-pelvic penetration pain cause personal distress and thus negatively affect the woman's and the couple's quality of life (Critelli *et al.*, 2016).

We have checked through clinical experience how effective an integrated approach can be in the treatment of dysfunctions due to sexual pain. The integrated approach allows having a holistic and non-fragmented view of the suffering person and offers a multi-causal aetiology of symptoms, thus providing a psychosomatic and somatopsychic interpretation of the disorder.

The therapeutic path includes the assessment to confirm the diagnosis and define a treatment protocol. Based on the disorder, the clients are administered both associated pharmacological therapy – if applicable – and rehabilitation physical therapy depending on their pelvic floor muscular tone. In both vaginismus and vulvodynia, in fact, it is possible to detect hypertonic pelvic muscles that interfere with the sexual activity (Critelli *et al.*, 2016).

In this context, Mark Grant's EMDR pain protocol has proved useful since the normalisation of the emotions connected to pain helps the client accept and manage them in a more effective way.

7.8   Rehabilitation intervention for sexual pain

If the pelvic floor muscles are hypertonic, the client is referred to a therapeutic path that includes different complementary phases and therapeutic directions.

The integrated treatment with EMDR includes a first preparation and stabilisation phase, aimed at creating/strengthening resources and at increasing body awareness through the following exercises:

- 'Safe place' protocol.
- 'Four elements' exercise to manage stress (Elan Shapiro).
- Respiratory training, relaxation exercises and body awareness and exercises to change dysfunctional respiratory patterns.
- Exercises to increase body awareness in general and the pelvic area in particular.

During the second phase of treatment, the goal is to reduce/eliminate pain and to reformulate the relationship with sexuality by the following:

- Processing some traumatic events connected to the perceived pain.
- Applying Mark Grant's EMDR pain protocol.
- Enhancing the experiential part with pelvic rehabilitator.

Depending on the diagnosis, during pelvic rehabilitation, the work earlier can be integrated with the following to enhance sexual functionality:

- Prescription of stretching exercises for the pelvic floor to perform at home.
- 8/10 biofeedback sessions.
- Some TENS (transcutaneous electrical nerve stimulation) sessions if required (Critelli *et al.*, 2016).

In fact, it has been proven that the rehabilitation part in the therapeutic course through biofeedback and TENS sessions, where required, represents a major step in terms of clinical effectiveness.

The main goal of this course is to improve the awareness and cortical representation of the muscles in the pelvic floor, thus increasing their perception by the client. Coming into contact and learning to know and perceive such muscles helps enhance the ability to control them voluntarily, which is a relevant aspect during sexual intercourse (Critelli *et al.*, 2016).

The need to care for the psychological aspect in these pathologies is self-evident, in full respect of the mind-body circular relationship. For this reason, the integrated approach encompasses both treatments focused on the body-muscular aspect and the EMDR treatment.

Following the completed path, clients have shown a substantial improvement in their muscular tone and in their vaginal habitability, with the following reduction in pain. The positive outcomes that emerged throughout the years in clinical practice have shown – in the view of an integrated approach – that the rehabilitation of the pelvic floor has been proven to be an effective ally in the treatment of disorders due to penetrative genital-pelvic pain.

Considering the person as a whole, in view of the individual's social-relational context, and in collaboration with different professionals, allows for an extremely effective clinical answer (Critelli *et al.*, 2016).

References

Ackerman, P.T., Newton, J.E.O., McPherson, W.B., Jones, J.G., Dykman, R.A. (1998), "Prevalence of posttraumatic stress disorder and other psychiatric diagnoses in three groups of abused children (sexual, physical, and both)", *Child Abuse and Neglect*, Vol. 22, pp. 759–774.

Alexander, P.C., Lupfer, S.R. (1987), "Family characteristics and long-term consequences associated with sexual abuse", *Archives of Sexual Behavior*, Vol. 16, pp. 235–245.

Almas, E., Landmark, B. (2010), "Non-pharmacological treatment of sexual problems, a review of research literature 1970–2008", *Sexologies*, Vol. 19, pp. 202–211.

Althof, S.E. (2000), "Psychological aspects of sexual dysfunction: The role of the couple", *International Journal of Impotence Research*, Vol. 12(S1), pp. S15–S20.

Althof, S.E. (2010), "What's new in sex therapy", *Journal of Sexual Medicine*, Vol. 7(1), pp. 5–13.

Althof, S.E., Leiblum, S.R. (2004), "Psychological and interpersonal dimensions of sexual function and dysfunction in sexual medicine", in *International Consultation on Sexual Dysfunctions*, Healt Publication, Paris.

American Psychiatric Association (1994), *Diagnostic and Statistical Manual of Mental Disorders. Fourth Edition*, American Psychiatric Association, Washington, DC.

American Psychiatric Association (2000), *Diagnostic and Statistical Manual of Mental Disorder. Fourth Edition*, Text Revision, Washington – Traduzione in italiano Andreoli, V., Cassano, G.B., Rossi, R. (ed.) (2002), *Manuale diagnostico e statistico dei disturbi mentali*, Masson, Milano.

American Psychiatric Association (2013), *Diagnostic and Statistical Manual of Mental Disorders. Fifth Edition (DSM-5)*, American Psychiatric Association, Washington – Traduzione in italiano (2014), *Manuale diagnostico e statistico dei disturbi mentali, Quinta edizione, DSM-5*, Masson, Milano.

Anda, R.F., Croft, J.B., Feliti, V.J., Nordenberg, D., Giles, W.H., Williamson, D.F., Giovino, G.A. (1999), "Adverse childhood experiences and smoking during adolescence and adulthood", *Journal of the American Medical Association*, Vol. 1(282), pp. 1652–1658.

Anda, R.F., Felitti, Y.J., Bremner, J.D., Walker, J.D., Whitfield, C., Perry, B.D., Dube, S.R., Giles, W.H. (2006), "The enduring effects of abuse and related adverse experiences in childhood: A convergence of evidence from neurobiology and epidemiology", *European Archives of Psychiatry and Clinical Neuroscience*, Vol. 256, pp. 174–186.

Andreasen, N.C., Pressler, M., Fox, M. (1977), "The scale for the assessment of positive symptoms (SAPS)", *Archives of General Psychiatry*, Vol. 34(2), pp. 215–220.

Aslan, D. (2008), "Psychosocial aspects of female sexual dysfunction: The importance of the couple's relationship", *Journal of Sexual Medicine*, Vol. 5(2), pp. 336–346.

Athanasiadis, L. (1998) "Premature ejaculation: Is it biogenic or psychogenic disorder?", *Sexual and Relationship Therapy*, Vol. 17(4), pp. 367–379.

Attili, G. (2011), "Trauma e relazione di coppia: il ruolo dell'attaccamento", in *Atti Congresso Nazionale EMDR, trauma e relazione*, Rome, Italy.

Aydin, S., Unal, D., Erol, H., Karaman, I., Yilmaz, Y., Sengul, E., Bayrakli, H. (2001), "Multicentral clinical evolution of the etiology of erectile dysfunction: A survey report", *International Urology and Nephrology*, Vol. 32, pp. 699–703.

Bagley, C., Wood, M., Young, L. (1994), "Victim to abuser: Mental health and behavioral sequels of child sexual abuse in a community survey of young adult males", *Child Abuse and Neglect*, Vol. 18, pp. 683–697.

Balbo, M. (2015), *Emdr e Disturbi dell'alimentazione. Tra passato, presente e futuro*, Giunti, Firenze.

Barker, R.T., Barker, S.T. (2007), "The use of EMDR in reducing presentation anxiety", *Journal of EMDR Practice and Research*, Vol. 1(2), pp. 100–108.

Basson, R. (2000), "The female sexual response: A different model", *Journal of Sex and Marital Therapy*, Vol. 26(1), pp. 1–16.

Basson, R. (2003), "Biopsychosocial models of women's sexual response: Applications to management of 'desire disorders'", *Sex Relationship Theory*, Vol. 18(1), pp. 107–115.

Basson, R. (2004), Women's sexual desire—Disordered or misunderstood?, *Journal of Sex & Marital Therapy*, Vol. 30(4), pp. 261–271.

Basson, R., Berman, J., Burnett, A., Derogatis, L., Ferguson, D., Fourcroy, J., Goldsten, I., Graziottin, A., Heiman, J., Laan, E., Leiblum, S.R., Padma-Nathan, H., Rosen, R.C., Segraves, K., Segraves, R.T., Shabsigh, R., Sipski, M., Wagner, G., Whipple, B. (2000), "Report of the international consensus development conference on female sexual dysfunction: Definitions and classifications", *Journal of Urology*, Vol. 163, pp. 888–893.

Basson, R., Leiblum, S.R., Brotto, L., Derogatis, L., Fourcroy, J., Fugl-Meyer, K., Graziottin, A., Heiman, J., Lann, E., Meston, C., Shover, L., van Lankveld, J., Weijmar Schultz, W. (2004), "Revised definitions of women's sexual dysfunction", *Journal of Sexual Medicine*, Vol. 1(1), pp. 40–48.

Basson, R., Leiblum, S.R., Brotto, L., Derogatis, L., Fourcroy, J., Fugl-Meyer, K., Graziottin, A., Heiman, J., Lann, E., Meston, C., van Lankveld, J., Weijmar Schultz, W. (2003), "Definitions of women's sexual dysfunction reconsidered: Advocating expansion and revision", *Journal of Psychosomatic Obstetrics & Gynecology*, Vol. 24(4), pp. 221–229.

Basson, R., Riley, A. (1994), "Vulvar vestibulitis syndrome: A common condition which may present as vaginismus", *Journal of Sex & Marital Therapy*, Vol. 9, pp. 221–224.

Bastianon, V., De Benedetti Gaddini, R. (1987), "Abuso e incuria verso l'infanzia", in Ferracuti, F. (ed.), *Trattato di criminologia, medicina criminologica e psichiatria forense, VI: Aspetti criminologici e psichiatrico-forensi dell'età minore*, Giuffrè, Milano, pp. 165–188.

Bavestrello, D., Piccini, F. (1991), "Benessere, malessere nella formazione del sessuologo". In *Atti del XXII Congresso degli Psicologi Italiani (SIPS)*, SIPS (Società Italiana di Psicologia), San Marino.

Becchi, M.A., Carulli, N. (2009), "Le basi scientifiche dell'approccio bio-psicosociale. Indicazione per l'acquisizione delle competenze mediche appropriate", *Medicina Italia*, Vol. 3, pp. 1–5.

Belkin, D.S., Greene, A.F., Rodrique, J.R., Boggs, S.R. (1994), "Psychopathology and history of sexual abuse", *Journal of Interpersonal Violence*, Vol. 9, pp. 535–547.

Bergler, E. (1951), *Counterfeit sex*, Grune & Stratton, New York, NY.

Berman, L.A., Berman, J.R., Chhabra, S., Goldstein, I. (2001), "Novel approaches to female sexual dysfunction", *Expert Opinion on Investigational Drugs*, Vol. 10, pp. 85–95.

Binik, Y.M. (2002), "Sexual dysfunction: A psychosocial perspective", in van der Kooy, J.H.H.M. (ed.), *Psychosocial Interventions for Sexual Dysfunctions*, Springer, New York, pp. 37–56.

Binik, Y.M. (2005), "The psychosocial aspects of sexual dysfunction", *Sexual and Relationship Therapy*, Vol. 20(2), pp. 155–169.

Binik, Y.M., Bergeron, S., Khalifè, S. (2000), "Dyspareunia", in Leiblum, S., Rosen, R. (eds.), *Principles and Practice of Sex Therapy*, Guilford Press, pp. 154–180.

Binik, Y.M., Reissing, E.D., Pukall, C.F. (2002), "The female sexual pain disorders: Genital pain or sexual dysfunction?", *Archives of Sexual Behavior*, Vol. 31, pp. 425–429.

Bisson, J. I., & Andrew M. (2007). Psychological treatment of post-traumatic stress disorder: A systematic review of randomized controlled trials. *Cochrane Database of Systematic Reviews,* 2007(3), CD003388. https://doi.org/10.1002/14651858.CD003388.pub3.

Bleustein, C., Tadir, Y., Hatzichristou, D. (2005), "The psychological aspects of sexual dysfunction: What can we learn from women?", *The Journal of Sexual Medicine*, Vol. 2(1), pp. 29–37.

Bloch, I. (1907), *Das sexualleben unserer Zeit in seinen Beziehungen zur modernen Kultur. (La vita sessuale del nostro tempo in relazione alla civiltà moderna)*, Marcus Verlagsbuchhandlung, Berlin.

Boccadoro, L., Carulli, S. (2008), *Il posto dell'amore negato. Sessualità e psicopatologie segrete*. Edizioni Tecnoprint, Ancona.

Bodie, J.A., Beeman, W.W., Monga, M. (2003), "Psychogenic erectile dysfunction", *International Journal of Psychiatry Medicine*, Vol. 33(3), pp. 273–293.

Bonierbale, M., Clement, A., Loundou, A., Simeoni, M.C., Barrau, K., Hamidi, K., Apter, M., Lancon, C., Auquier, P. (2006), "A new evaluation concept and its measurement: Male sexual anticipating cognitions", *Journal of Sexual Medicine*, Vol. 3, pp. 96–103.

Books (1983), *Traduzione in italiano: Attaccamento e perdita. Vol. 3: La perdita della madre*, Boringhieri, Torino.

Boon, S., Draijer, N. (1993). "Dissociation and the treatment of trauma." In M.P. Dezwart Abrams (Ed.), *Trauma and Dissociation: A Handbook for Clinicians* (pp. 183–202). New York: Wiley.

Brand, E.F., King, C.A., Olson, E., Ghaziuddin, N., Naylor, M. (1996), "Depressed adolescents with a history of sexual abuse: Diagnostic comorbidity and suicidality", *Child Adolescence Psychiatry*, Vol. 35(1), pp. 34–41.

Bray, M. (1994). "Child sexual abuse, family life and the Children Act." In A. Levy (Ed.), *Re-Focus on Child Abuse* (pp. 59–72). London, UK: Hawksmere PLC.

Breslau, N., Chilcoat, H.D., Kessler, R.C., Peterson, E.L., Lucia, V.C. (1999), "Vulnerability to assaultive violence: Further specification of sex difference in post-traumatic stress disorder", *Psychology and Medicine*, Vol. 29, pp. 813–821.

Breslau, N., Davis, G., Andreski, P. (1995), "Risk factors for PTSD-related traumatic events: A prospective analysis", *American Journal of Psychiatry*, Vol. 152, pp. 529–535.

Brewin, C.R., Andrews, B., Valentine, J.D. (2000), "Meta-analysis of risk factors for post-traumatic stress disorder in trauma-exposed adults", *Journal of Consulting and Clinical Psychology*, Vol. 68, pp. 748–766.

Briere, J., Evans, D., Runtz Wall, T. (1988), "Symptomatology in men who were molested as children: A comparison study", *American Journal of Orthopsychiatry*, Vol. 58, pp. 457–461.

Brown, K.W., McGoldrick, T., Buchanan, R. (1997), "Body dysmorphic disorder: Seven cases treated with eye movement desensitization and reprocessing", *Behavioural and Cognitive Psychotherapy*, Vol. 25(2), pp. 203–207.

Brown, S., Shapiro, F. (2006), "EMDR in the treatment of borderline personality disorder", *Clinical Case Studies*, Vol. 5, pp. 403–420.

Browne, A., Finkelhor, D. (1986), *A Sourcebook on Child Sexual Abuse*, Sage Publications, Beverly Hills.

Browning, C. (1999), "Floatback and float forward: Techniques for linking past, present and future", *EMDRIA Newsletter*, Vol. 4(3), pp. 12, 34.

Burchardt, M., Burchardt, T., Anastasiadis, A.G. (2002), "Sexual dysfunction is common and overlooked in female patients with hypertension", *Journal of Sex & Marital Therapy*, Vol. 28, pp. 17–26.

Burgess, A.W., Holmstrom, L.L. (1974), "Rape trauma syndrome", *American Journal of Psychology*, Vol. 9, pp. 981–986.

Burns, B.J., Hoagwood, K., Maultsby, L.T., Epstein, M.H., Kutash, K., Duchnowski, A. (1998), "Improving outcomes for children and adolescents with serious emotional and behavioral disorders: Current and future directions", in Epstein, M., Kutash, K., Duchnowski, A. (eds.), *Outcomes for Children and Youth with Emotional and Behavioral Disorders and Their Families: Programs and Evaluation Best Practices*, Pro-Ed, Austin, TX, pp. 685–707.

Busato, W., Galindo, C.C. (2004), "Topical anaesthetic use for treating premature ejaculation: A double-blind, randomized, placebo-controlled study", *International Journal of Impotence Research*, Vol. 93(7), pp. 1018–1021.

Canepa, G. (1987), "Il maltrattamento dei minori", in Ferracuti, F. (ed.), *Trattato di criminologia, medicina criminologica e psichiatria forense, VI: Aspetti criminologici e psichiatrico-forensi dell'età minore*, Giuffrè, Milano, pp. 151–164.

Carani, C., Isidori, A.M., Granata, A., Carosa, E., Maggi, M., Lenzi, A., Jannini, E.A. (2005, December 1), "Multicenter study on the prevalence of sexual symptoms in male hypo- and hyperthyroid patients", *Journal of Clinical Endocrinology and Metabolism*, Vol. 90(12), pp. 6472–6479.

Carlson, C.R., Rucker, R.R., Johnson, C. (2000), "Sexual dysfunction in chronic pain patients: A review of the literature", *Journal of Sex & Marital Therapy*, Vol. 26(4), pp. 355–364.

Carlson, E.B. (1997), *Trauma Assessments: A Clinician's Guide*, Guildford, New York.

Carlson, E.B., Dalenberg, C. (2000), "A conceptual framework for the impact of traumatic experiences", *Trauma, Violence and Abuse*, Vol. 1, pp. 4–28.

Carvalho, J.C.G.R., Agualusa, L.M., Moreira, L.M.R., Costa, J.C. (2014), "Multimodal therapeutic approach of vaginismus: An innovative approach through trigger point infiltration and pulsed radiofrequency of the pudendal nerve", *Brazilian Journal of Anesthesiology*, pp. 1–5.

Cayan, S., Bozlu, M., Canpolat, B., Akbay, E. (2004), "The assessment of sexual functions in women with male partner complaining of erectile dysfunction: Does treatment of male sexual dysfunction improve female partner's sexual functions?", *Journal of Sex and Marital Therapy*, Vol. 30, pp. 333–341.

Chevret, M., Jaudinot, E., Sullivan, K., Marrel, A., De Gendre, A.S. (2004), "Impact of erectile dysfunction (ED) on sexual life of female partner: Assessment with the index of sexual life (ISL) questionnaire", *Journal of Sex and Marital Therapy*, Vol. 30, pp. 157–172.

Cohen, S., Janicki, D., McDaniel, B. (2000), "The role of psychosocial factors in sexual dysfunction", *Archives of Sexual Behavior*, Vol. 29(4), pp. 367–373.

Collings, S.J. (1995), "The long-term effects of contact and noncontact forms of child sexual abuse in a sample of university men", *Child Abuse and Neglect*, Vol. XX(5), pp. 447–455.

Cook, A., Spinazzola, J., Ford, J., Lanktree, C., Blaustein, M., Cloitre, M., van der Kolk, B. (2005), "Complex trauma in children and adolescents", *Psychiatric Annals*, Vol. 35, pp. 390–398.

Copeland, W.E., Keeler, G., Angold, A., Costello, E.J. (2007), "Traumatic events and post-traumatic stress in childhood", *Archives of General Psychiatry*, Vol. 64, pp. 577–584.

Cosentino, C.E., Meyer-Bahlburg, H.F.L., Alpert, J.L., Weinberg, S.L., Gaines, R. (1995), "Sexual behavior problems and psychopathology symptoms in sexually abused girls", *Journal of American Academic Child Adolescence Psychiatry*, Vol. 34(8), pp. 1033–1042.

Critelli, C., Iasevoli, M., Tripodi, F. (2016), "Intervento riabilitativo per il dolore sessuale", *Rivista di Sessuologia Clinica*, Vol. 1, pp. 79–81.

Cross, T.P., De Vos, E., Whitcomb, D. (1994), "Prosecution of child sexual abuse: Which cases accepted?", *Child Abuse and Neglect*, Vol. 18(8), pp. 661–677.

Crowe, M.J., Gillan, P., Golombok, S. (1981), "Form and content in the conjoint treatment of sexual dysfunction: A controlled study", *Behaviour Research and Therapy*, Vol. 19(1), pp. 47–54.

D'Andrea, W., Ford, J., Stolbach, B., Spinazzola, J. (2015), "Comprendere il trauma interpersonale nei bambini: perché abbiamo bisogno di una diagnosi orientata allo sviluppo", *Quaderni Infanzia e Adolescenza*, Vol. 14(1), pp. 61–82.

D'Ario, D. (2015), *Dolore pelvico cronico*, Facoltà di Medicina e Chirurgia, Napoli, p. 12.

Darves-Bornoz, J.M., Lèpine, I.P., Choquet, M., Berger, C., Degiovanni, A., Gaillard, P. (1998), "Predictive factors of chronic post-traumatic stress disorder in rape victims", *European Psychiatry*, Vol. 13, pp. 281–287.

De Jongh, A., Ten Broeke, E., Renssen, M.R. (1999), "Treatment of specific phobias with eye movement desensitization and reprocessing: Protocol, empirical status, and conceptual issues", *Journal of Anxiety Disorders*, Vol. 13(1–2), pp. 69–85.

De Jongh, A., van den Oord, H.J.M., Ten Broeke, E. (2002), "Efficacy of eye movement desensitization and reprocessing in the treatment of specific phobias: Four single-case studies on dental phobia", *Journal of Clinical Psychology*, Vol. 58(12), pp. 1489–1503.

De Leo, D., Kilmartin, C. (1999), "Sexual dysfunction in men: A review of the literature", *Archives of Sexual Behavior*, Vol. 28(1), pp. 23–35.

De Leo, G., Petruccelli, I. (1999), *L'abuso sessuale infantile e la pedofilia*, Franco Angeli, Milano.

de Roos, C., Veenstra, A.C., de Jongh, A., den Hollander-Gijsman, M.E., van der Wee, N.J.A., Zitman, F.G., van Rood, Y.R. (2010), "Treatment of chronic phantom limb pain using a trauma-focused psychological approach", *Pain Research & Management*, Vol. 15(2), pp. 65–71.

De Young, M. (1982), *The Sexual Victimization of Children*, McFarland & Co., London.

Dennerstein, L. (2006), "Well-being, symptoms and the menopausal transition", *Maturitas*, Vol. 54(1), pp. 14–23.

Dennerstein, L., Koochaki, P.E., Barton, I. (2006), "Hypoactive sexual desire disorder in menopausal women: A survey of Western European women", *Journal of Sexual Medicine*, Vol. 3(2), pp. 212–222.

Dent, B.K. (1993), "Child sexual abuse: Problems for adults survivors", *Journal of Mental Health*, Vol. 2(4), pp. 329–338.

Dèttore, D. (2001), *Psicologia e psicopatologia del comportamento sessuale*, McGraw-Hill, Milano.

Diamond, M. (1965), "A critical evaluation of the ontogeny of human sexual behavior", *Quarterly Review of Biology*, Vol. 40, pp. 147–175.

Dinsmore, W.W. (2005, May), "Patient-acquired hepatitis B and HIV following erectile dysfunction therapy", *International Journal of STD & AIDS*, Vol. 16(5), pp. 390–391.

Draijer, N. (1990), *Seksuele traumatisering in de jeugd: gevolgen op lange termijn van seksueel misbruik van meisjes door verwanten*, Sua, Amsterdam.

Draijer, N., Boon, S. (1999), "The imitation of dissociative identità disorder: Patients at risk, therapist at risk", *Journal of Psychiatry & Law*, Vol. 11, pp. 301–322.

Draijer, N., Laan, E. (1999), "Sexual dysfunction in women with a history of sexual abuse: A review", *Journal of Sex & Marital Therapy*, Vol. 25(2), pp. 125–133.

Dube, S.R., Anda, R.F., Felitti, V.J., Chapman, D.P., Williamson, D.F., Giles, W.H. (2001), "Childhood abuse, household dysfunction and the risk of attempted suicide throughout the life span: Findings from the adverse childhood experiences study", *Journal of the American Medical Association*, Vol. 286, pp. 3089–3096.

Dube, S.R., Felitti, V.J., Dong, M., Chapman, D.P., Giles, W.H., Anda, R.E. (2003), "Childhood abuse, neglect, and household dysfunction and the risk of illicit drug use: The adverse childhood experiences study", *Pediatrics*, Vol. 111, pp. 564–572.

Duenas, J.M. (1986), "Sexual dysfunction: A review of the literature", *Archives of Sexual Behavior*, Vol. 15(5), pp. 425–438.

Dworkin, E.R. (2005), "Sexual assault victimization and the psychological consequences: A review of the literature", *Journal of Trauma & Dissociation*, Vol. 6(4), pp. 57–71.

Dworkin, M. (2010), *La relazione terapeutica nel trattamento EMDR*, Raffaello Cortina Editore, Milano.

Emily, J.O., Best, S.R., Lipsey, T.L., Weiss, D.S. (2003), "Predictors of post-traumatic stress disorder and symptoms in adults: A meta-analysis", *Psychological Bulletin*, Vol. 129, pp. 52–73.

Engel, G.L. (1977), "The need for a new medical model: A challenge for biomedicine", *Science*, Vol. 196(4286), pp. 129–136.

Engel, G.L. (1997), "The need for a new medical model: A challenge for biomedicine", *Science*, Vol. 196(4286), pp. 129–136.

Eulenburg, A. (1978), *Lehrbuch der Nervenkrankheiten*, August Hirschwald, Berlin.

Faretta, E. (2014), *Trauma e Malattia. L'EMDR in Psiconcologia*, Mimesis, Milano.

Farina, B., Imperatori, C., Quintiliani, I., Castelli Gattinara, P., Onofri, A., Lepore, M., Brunetti, R., Losurdo, A., Testani, E., Della Marca, G. (2014), "Neurophysiological correlates of eye movement desensitization and reprocessing sessions: Preliminary evidence for traumatic memories integration", *Clinical Physiology and Functional Imaging*, pp. 1–9.

Farina, B., Mazzotti, E., Pasquini, P., Mantione, M.G. (2011), "Somatoform and psychoform dissociation among women with orgasmic and sexual pain disorders", *Journal of Trauma & Dissociation*, Vol. 12(5).

Fedele, D., Coscelli, C., Cucinotto, D., Forti, G., Santeusanio, F., Fiori, G., Velona, T., Lavezzari, M. (2001), "Management of erectile dysfunction in diabetic subjects: Results from a survey of 400 centres in Italy", *Diabetes, Nutrition & Metabolism*, Vol. 14(5), pp. 277–282.

Felitti, V.J., Anda, R.F., Nordenberg, D., Williamson, D.F., Spitz, A.M., Edwards, V., Koss, M.P., Marks, J.S. (1998), "Relationship of childhood abuse and household dysfunction to many the leading causes of death in adults; The adverse childhood experiences, ACE study 14", *American Journal of Preventive Medicine*, Vol. 14, pp. 245–258.

Fenwick, P. (1994), "Psychological aspects of sexual dysfunction in women", *Journal of Family Planning and Reproductive Health Care*, Vol. 20(2), pp. 64–68.

Fernandez, I., Faretta, E. (2007), "Eye movement desensitization and reprocessing in the treatment of panic disorder with Agorophobia", *Clinical Case Studies*, Vol. 6, pp. 44–63.

Fernandez, I., Maslovaric, G., Veniero Galvagni, M.V. (2011), *Traumi psicologici, ferite dell'anima. Il contributo della terapia con EMDR*, Liguori, Napoli.

Finkelhor, D. (1990), "Early and long-term effects of child sexual abuse: An update", *Professional Psychology: Research and Practice*, Vol. 21(5), pp. 325–330.

Finkelhor, D. (2008), *Childhood victimization*, Oxford University Press, New York.

Finkelhor, D., Baron, L. (1986), "Risk factors for child sexual abuse", *Journal of Interpersonal Violence*, Vol. 1(1), pp. 43–71.

Finkelhor, D., Ormrod, R.K., Turner, H.A. (2009), "Lifetime assessment of poly-victimization in a national sample of children and youth", *Child Abuse and Neglect*, Vol. 33, pp. 403–411.

Foa, E.B., Zinbarg, R., Rothbaum, B.O. (1992), "Uncontrollability and unpredictability in post-traumatic stress disorder: An animal model", *Psychological Bulletin*, Vol. 112, pp. 218–238.

Fosha, D. (2016), *Il potere trasformativo delle emozioni*, ISC, Sassari.

Franzese, R. (2015), "Ruolo della riabilitazione del pavimento pelvico nel trattamento dei disturbi sessuali femminili caratterizzati dal dolore", in *Facoltà di Medicina e Chirurgia*, Napoli, pp. 47–51.

Fraser, G.A. (1991), "The dissociative table technique: A strategy for working with ego states in dissociative disorders and ego state therapy", *Dissociation*, Vol. 4(4), pp. 205–213.

Fraser, G.A. (2003), "Fraser's dissociative table technique revisited, revised: A strategy for working with ego states in dissociative disorders and ego-state therapy", *Journal of Trauma and Dissociation*, Vol. 4(4), pp. 5–28.

Freyd, J.J. (1996), *Betrayal Trauma: The Logic of Forgetting Childhood Trauma*, Harvard University Press, Cambridge, USA.

Friedman, M. (1973), "Success phobia and retarded ejaculation", *American Journal of Psychotherapy*, Vol. 1, pp. 766–775.

Friedrich, W.N., Schaefer, C. (1995), "Sexual dysfunctions in children and adolescents: Clinical issues and treatment approaches", *Journal of Child Sexual Abuse*, Vol. 4(2), 1–23.

Fromuth, M.E. (1986), "The relationship of childhood sexual abuse with later psychological and sexual adjustment in a sample of college women", *Child Abuse and Neglect*, Vol. 10, pp. 5–15.

Fromuth, M.E., Burkhart, B.R. (1989), "Long-term psychological correlates of childhood sexual abuse in two samples of college men", *Child Abuse and Neglect*, Vol. 13, pp. 533–542.

Fulceri, F., Rondinelli, S., Spennato, R., Speranza, B., Viccaro, M.C., Vitello, S. (2016), "L'approccio gestaltico analitico alla sessualità", in *Disturbi sessuali e psicoterapia, Psicobiettivo, N. 2*, FrancoAngeli, Milano.

Fullerton, D.T., Wonderlich, S.A., Gosnell, B.A. (1995), "Clinical characteristics of eating disorder patient who report sexual or physical abuse", *International Journal of Eating Disorders*, Vol. 17(3), pp. 243–249.

Gallo, L.C., Fortmann, A.L., Kauffman, M. (2010), "Sexual functioning in women with heart disease: A review of the literature", *Journal of Sex & Marital Therapy*, Vol. 36(2), pp. 152–164.

Gauvreau, P., Bouchard, S. (2008), "Preliminary evidence for the efficacy of EMDR in treating generalized anxiety disorder", *Journal of EMDR Practice and Research*, Vol. 2(1), pp. 26–40.

George, C., Kaplan, N., Main, M. (1984, 1985, 1996), "The adult attachment interview", Unpublished Manuscript, University of California at Berkeley.

Glaser, D. (2000), "Child abuse and neglect and the brain: A review", *Journal of Child Psychology and Psychiatry*, Vol. 41, pp. 97–116.

Goldstein, A.J., Beurs, E., Chambless, D.L. (2000), "EMDR for panic disorder with agoraphobia: Comparison with waiting list and credible attention-placebo control conditions", *Journal of Consulting & Clinical Psychology*, Vol. 68(6), pp. 947–956.

Goldstein, I., Berman, J.R. (1998), "Vasculogenic female sexual dysfunction. Vaginal engorgement and clitoral erectile insufficiency syndromes", *International Journal of Impotence*, Vol. 10, pp 584–590.

Gomez, A.M. (2013), *EMDR Therapy and Adjunct Approaches with Children*, Sprinter Publishing Company, New York.

Gonzalez Vazquez, A. (2013), *I disturbi dissociativi. Diagnosi e trattamento*, Giovanni Fioriti Editore, Roma.

Gonzalez Vazquez, A., Mosquera, D. (2012), *EMDR and Dissociation: The Progressive Approach*, Amazon Imprint, Charleston, SC.

Grant, M. (2023), *Pain Control with EMDR: Treatment Manual, Eighth Revised Edition*, Trauma and Pain Management Services Pty Ltd, ISBN: 9781925457445(AbeBooks) (ThriftBooks).

Grant, M., Threlfo, C. (2002), "EMDR in the treatment of chronic pain", *Journal of Clinical Psychology*, Vol. 58(12), pp. 1505–1520.

Graziottin, A. (2007), "Prevalence and evalutation of sexual health problems HSDD in Europe", *Journal of Sexual Medicine*, Vol. 4(3), pp. 211–219.

Green, A.H. (1994), "La violenza sessuale infantile: conseguenze immediate e a lungo termine e loro trattamento", *Terapia Familiare*, Vol. 46, pp. 15–35.

Greenwald, E., Leitnberg, H., Cado, S., Tartan, M.J. (1990), "Childhood sexual abuse: Long-term effects on psychological and sexual functioning in a nonclinical and nonstudent sample of adult women", *Child Abuse and Neglect*, Vol. 14, pp. 503–513.

Hafez, E.S., Hafez, S.D. (2005, January–February), "Erectile dysfunction: Anatomical parameters, etiology, diagnosis and therapy", *Archives of Andrology*, Vol. 51(1), pp. 15–31.

Hall, K., Hall, M. (1989), "The role of psychosexual factors in the etiology of erectile dysfunction: A review", *Journal of Sex Research*, Vol. 26(2), pp. 218–231.

Hanks, H., Hobbs, C., Sonne, J.L., Woods, L.R. (1988), "Early signs and recognition of sexual abuse in the pre-school child", in Browne, K., Davies, C., Stratton, P. (eds.), *Early, Prediction and Prevention of Child Abuse*, John Wiley & Sons, London, pp. 139–160.

Harrar, M.A., Hays, R.D., Ickovics, J.R. (1999), "Sexual function in a community sample of women: The role of depression and anxiety", *Journal of Sex Research*, Vol. 36(2), pp. 112–118.

Harrar, S., Vantine, J. (1999), *Extraordinary Togetherness: A Woman's Guide to Love, Sex and Intimacy*, Rodale Press, Emmaus, PA.

Hartmann, U., Shedlowski, M., Kruger, T.H.C. (2005), "Cognitive and partner-related factors in rapid ejaculation: Differences between dysfunctional men", *World Journal of Urology*, Vol. 23, pp. 93–101.

Hawton, K. (1985), *Sex Therapy. A Practical Guide*, Oxford University Press, New York – Traduzione in italiano (1987), *Guida pratica alla terapia sessuale*, Astrolabio, Roma.

Heiman, J.R. (1998), "Psychophysiological models of female sexual response", *International Journal of Impotence Research*, Vol. 10, pp. 94–97.

Heiman, J.R. (2000), "Orgasmic disorders in women", in Leiblum, S., Rosen, R. (eds.), *Principles and Practice of Sex Therapy*, Guildford Press, New York, pp. 118–153.

Helgason, A.R., Adolfsson, J., Dickman, P., Arver, S., Fredrikson, M., Gothberg, M., Steineck, G. (1996), "Sexual desire, erection, orgasm and ejaculatory functions and their importance to elderly Swedish men: A population-based study", *Age and Ageing*, Vol. 25(4), pp. 285–291.

Hendrickx, L., Gijs, L., Enzlin, P. (2013), "Distress, sexual dysfunctions, and DSM: Dialogue at cross purposes?", *Journal of Sexual Medicine*, Vol. 10(3), pp. 630–641.

Herman, J.L. (1981), *Father-Daughter Incest*, Harvard University Press, Cambridge.

Herman, J.L. (1992), "Complex PTDS: A syndrome in survivors of prolonged and repeated trauma", *Journal of Traumatic Stress*, Vol. 5(3), pp. 377–391.

Herman, J.L., Perry, J.C., van Der Kolk, B.A. (1989), "Childhood trauma in borderline personalità disorder", *American Journal of Psychiatry*, Vol. 146, pp. 490–495.

Hesse, E. (1999), "The adult attachment interview: Historical and current perspectives", in Cassidy, J., Shaker, P.R. (eds.), *Handbook of Attachment: Theory, Research and Clinical Applications*, The Guildford Press, New York, pp. 395–433.

Hillis, S.D., Anda, R.F., Dube, S.R., Felitti, V.J., Marchbanks, P.A., Marks, J.S. (2004), "The association between adverse childhood experiences and adolescent pregnancy, long-term psychosocial consequences, and fetal death", *Pediatrics*, Vol. 113, pp. 320–327.

Hirsch, M. (1998), "Functional neurovascular anatomy", Presented at the Boston University School of Medicine and the Department of Urology Conference: New Perspectives in the Management of Female Sexual Dysfunction, Burlington, MA.

Hite, S. (1998), "The female orgasm and women today", in Simonelli, C., Petruccelli, F., Vizzari, V. (eds.), *Sessualità e terzo millennio*, Franco Angeli, Milano.

Holbrook, T.L., Hoyt, D.B., Stein, M.B., Sieber, W.J. (2002), "Gender differences in long-term post-traumatic disorder outcomes after major trauma. Women are at higher risk of aderse outcomes that men", *Journal of Trauma*, Vol. 53, pp. 882–888.

Holmes, J. (1998), "The search for the secure base: Attachment theory and psychotherapy", *The Psychoanalytic Review*, Vol. 85(3), pp. 551–563.

Hughes, D. (2012), "La comunicazione delle emozioni e lo sviluppo dell'autonomia e dell'intimità all'interno della terapia familiare", in Fosha, D., Siegel, D., Solomon, M. (eds.), *Attraversare le emozioni. Nuovi modelli di psicoterapia. Vol. 2*, Mimesis, Milano-Udine.

Irwin, H.J. (1998, February), "Affective predictors of dissociation. II: Shame and guilt", *Journal of Clinical Psychology*, Vol. 54(2), pp. 237–245.

Jackson, G., Betteridge, J., Dean, J., Eardley, I., Hall, R., Holdright, D., Holmes, S., Kirby, M., Riley, A., Sever, P. (2002), "A systematic approach to erectile dysfunction in the cardiovascular patient: A consensus statement-update 2002", *International Journal of Clinical Practice*, Vol. 56(9), pp. 631, 663–671.

Jannini, E.A., Lenzi, A. (2005), "Ejaculatory disorders: Epidemiology and current approaches to definition, classification and subtyping", *World Journal of Urology*, Vol. 23, pp. 68–75.

Jannini, E.A., Maggi, M., Lenzi, A. (2011), "Evaluation of premature ejaculation", *Journal of Sexual Medicine*, Vol. 8, pp. 328–334.

Jannini, E.A., Simonelli, C., Lenzi, A. (2002a), "Disorders of ejaculation", *Journal of Endocrinological Investigation*, Vol. 25, pp. 1006–1019.

Jannini, E.A., Simonelli, C., Lenzi, A. (2002b), "Sexological approach to ejaculatory dysfunction", *International Journal of Andrology*, Vol. 25, pp. 1–7.

Jehu, D. (1988), *Beyond Sexual Abuse. Therapy with Women Who Were Childhood Victims*, John Wiley & Sons, Chichester.

Johnson, S.M., Whiffen, V. (2003), "Attachment processes in couple and family therapy", in Cutrona, J.L., Johnson, S.M., Whiffen, V. (eds.), *Couple and Family Therapy: A Therapist's Guide to Theoretical Models and Interventions*. Guilford Press, New York, pp. 123–148.

Jurich, J.A., Myers-Bowman, K.S. (1998), "Systems theory and its application to research on human sexuality", *Journal of Sex Research*, Vol. 35(1), pp. 72–87.

Kamischke, A., Nieschlag, E. (2002), "Update on medical treatment of ejaculatory disorders", *International Journal of Andrology*, Vol. 25, pp. 333–344.

Kaplan, H.S. (1974), *The New Sex Therapy*, Brunner/Mazel, New York – Traduzione in italiano (1976), *Nuove terapie sessuali*, Bompiani, Milano.

Kaplan, H.S. (1982), *The New Sex Therapy: Active Treatment for Sexual Dysfunction*, Simon & Schuster, New York.

Kaplan, H.S. (1979), *Disorders of Sexual desire*, Brunner/Mazel, New York – Traduzione in italiano (1981), *I disturbi del desiderio sessuale*, Mondadori, Milano.

Kardiner, A., Spiegel, J.P. (1947), *Trauma and the American Soldier*, Government Printing Office, Washington, DC.

Kigozi, G., Wawer, M.J., Ndinya-Achola, J. (2008), "The relationship between sexual dysfunction and quality of life in HIV-infected men in Uganda", *The Journal of Sexual Medicine*, Vol. 5(4), pp. 1037–1044.

Kim, S.C., Pang, K. (2006), "The impact of erectile dysfunction on quality of life: A cross-sectional study in a Korean population", *The Journal of Sexual Medicine*, Vol. 3(3), pp. 413–419.

Kim, S.C., Seo, K.K. (1998), "Efficacy and safety of fluoxetine, sertraline and clomipramine in patients with premature ejaculation: A double-blind, placebo controlled study", *Journal of Urology*, Vol. 159, pp. 425–427.

Kirana, S.P., Tripodi, F., Reisman, Y., Porst, H. (2013), *The EFS and ESSM. Syllabus of Clinical Sexology*, Medix, Amsterdam.

Kirby, M., Jackson, G., Simonsen, U. (2005), "Endothelial dysfunction links erectile dysfunction to heart disease", *International Journal of Clinical Practice*, Vol. 59(2), pp. 225–259.

Kiser, L.J., Ackerman, B.J., Brown, E., Edwards, B.N., McColgan, E., Pugh, R., Pruitt, B.D. (1988), "Post-traumatic stress disorder in young children: A reaction to purported sexual abuse", *Journal of the American Academy of Child and Adolescent Psychiatry*, Vol. 27(5), pp. 645–650.

Klein, R., Klein, B.E., Moss, S.E. (2005), "Ten-year incidence of self-reported erectile dysfunction in people with long-term type 1 diabetes", *Journal of Diabetes and its Complications*, Vol. 19(1), pp. 35–41.

Knipe, J. (2017), *EMDR Toolbox. Teoria e trattamento del PTSD complesso e della dissociazione*, Giovanni Fioriti Editore, Roma.

Knopf, J., Seiler, M. (1993), *Quando il sesso dorme*, Sperling & Kupfer, Milano.

Knopf, R.A., Hurst, M.W., McCarthy, B. (1993), "The role of sexual dysfunction in the marital relationship: A review of the literature", *Journal of Sex & Marital Therapy*, Vol. 19(1), pp. 25–34.

Koch, M. (1980), "Sexual abuse in children", *Adolescence*, Vol. 15(59), pp. 643–648.

Korn, D.L., Leeds, A.M. (2002), "Preliminary evidence of efficacy for EMDR resource development and installation in the stabilization phase of treatment of complex posttraumatic stress disorder", *Journal of Clinical Psychology*, Vol. 58(12), pp. 1465–1487.

Krakow, B., Tandberg, D., Barey, M., Scriggins, L. (1995), "Nightmares and sleep disturbance in sexually assaulted women", *Dreaming Journal of the Association for the Study of Dreams*, Vol. 5(3), pp. 199–206.

Lamprecht, F., Kohnke, C., Lempa, W., Sack, M., Matzke, M., Munte, T. (2004), "Event-related potentials and EMDR treatment of post-traumatic stress disorder", *Neuroscience Research*, Vol. 49, pp. 267–272.

Lansing, K., Amen, D.G., Hanks, C., Rudy, L. (2005), "High resolution brain SPECT imaging and EMDR in police officers with PTSD", *Journal of Neuropsychiatry and Clinical Neurosciences*, Vol. 17, pp. 526–532.

Laumann, E.O., Nicolosi, A., Glasser, D.B., Paik, A., Ginger, C., Moreira, E., Wang, T. (2005), "Sexual problems among women and men aged 40–80 years: Prevalence and correlates identified in the global studies of sexual attitudes and behaviors", *International Journal of Impotent Research*, Vol. 17, pp. 39–57.

Laumann, E.O., Paik, A., Rosen, R.C. (1999), "Sexual dysfunction in the United States: Relevance and predictors", *JAMA*, Vol. 281, pp. 573–544.

Lazarus, A.E. (1963), "The treatment of chronic frigidità by sistematic desensitization", *Journal of Nervous and Mental Disease*, Vol. 136, pp. 272–278.

Leeds, A. M., & Shapiro, F. (2000). EMDR and resource installation: Principles and procedures for enhancing current functioning and resolving traumatic experiences. In J. Carlson & L. Sperry (Eds.), *Brief therapy with individuals & couples* (pp. 469–534). Zeig, Tucker & Theisen.

Leiblum, S.R. (2002), "Reconsidering gender differences in sexual desire: An update", *Sexual and Relationship Therapy*, Vol. 17(1), pp. 57–68.

Leiblum, S.R. (2007), *Principles and Practices of Sex Therapy. Fourth Edition*, Guildford Press, New York.

Leiblum, S.R., Graziottin, A. (2004), "Classificazione dei disturbi sessuali femminili, nuove prospettive", in Rosen, R.C., Leiblum, S.R., Graziottin, A. (eds.), *Principi e pratica di terapia sessuale*, CIC Edizioni Internazionali, Roma, pp. 115–124.

Leiblum, S.R., Rosen, R. (2000), *Principles and Practice of Sex Therapy*, Guildford Press, New York.

Leiblum, S.R., Rosen, R.C., D'Agostino, J. (2000), "Assessment of female sexual dysfunction: A review of the literature", *Journal of Sexual Medicine*, Vol. 1(1), pp. 121–127.

Leskela, J., Dieperink, M., Thuras, P. (2002, June), "Shame and post-traumatic stress disorder", *Journal Trauma Stress*, Vol. 15(3), pp. 223–226.

Levin, P., Lazrove, S., van der Kolk, B.A. (1999), "What psychological testing and neuroimaging tell us about the treatment of posttraumatic stress disorder (PTSD) by eye movement desensibilization and reprocessing", *Journal of Anxiety Disorders*, Vol. 13, pp. 159–172.

Levine, L.A. (2000), "Diagnosis and treatment of erectile dysfunction", *The American Journal of Medicine*, Vol. 18(109), Suppl. 9 A, pp. S–12 S, discussion 29, pp. S–30 S.

Levine, S.B. (2003), "The nature of sexual desire", *Archives of Sexual Behavior*, Vol. 32(3), pp. 279–285.

Levine, S.B., Landon, H.M. (2002), "The role of sexual functioning in the evaluation and treatment of male erectile dysfunction", *Journal of Sexual Medicine*, Vol. 1(1), pp. 45–56.

Lewis, R.H., Fugl-Meyer, K.S. (2004), "Definition, classification and epidemiology of sexual dysfunction", in Lue, T.F., Basson, R., Rosen, R.C. (eds.), *Sexual Medicine, Sexual Dysfunction in Men and in Women, International Consultation on Sexual Dysfunctions*, Health Pubblication, Paris.

Lief, H. (1997), "Inhibited sexual desire", *Medical Aspects of Human Sexuality*, Vol. 11, pp. 94–95.

Liotti, G., Farina, B. (2000), "The role of attachment in the development of trauma: Implications for the treatment of post-traumatic stress disorder", *Clinical Psychology & Psychotherapy*, Vol. 7(3), pp. 137–146.

Liotti, G., Farina, B. (2011), *Sviluppi traumatici. Eziopatogenesi, clinica e terapia della dimensione dissociativa*, Raffaello Cortina Editore, Milano.

Lisak, D. (1994), "The psychological impact of sexual abuse: Content analysis of interviews with males survivors", *Journal of Traumatic Stress*, Vol. 7, pp. 525–548.

Lisak, D. (1997), *Sexual Abuse of Males: Prevalente, Lasting Effects and Resources*, www.jimhopper.com/.

Lo Piccolo, J. (1985), "Diagnosis and treatment of male sexual dysfunction", *Journal of Sex and Marital Therapy*, Vol. 11, pp. 215–232.

Lombardo, F., Sgro, P., Grandini, L., Dondero, F., Jannini, E.A., Lenzi, A. (2004, October), "Might erectile dysfunction be due to the thermolabile variant of methylenetetrahydrofolate reductase?", *Journal of Endocrinological Investigation*, Vol. 27(99), pp. 883–885.

Luber, M. (2015), *I protocolli terapeutici dell'EMDR. Condizioni di base e specifiche*, Giovanni Fioriti Editore, Roma.

Lue, T.F. (2001, October), "Neurogenic erectile dysfunction", *Clinical Autonomic Research*, Vol. 11(5), pp. 285–294.

Luzzi, L., Law, S. (2006), "A qualitative study of sexual dysfunction in men with multiple sclerosis", *International Journal of MS Care*, Vol. 8(2), pp. 67–72.

Lynch, M. (1988), "The consequences of child abuse", in Browne, K., Davies, C., Stratton, P. (eds.), *Early Prediction and Prevention of Child Abuse*, John Wiley & Sons, London, pp. 202–212.

Malagoli Togliatti, M., Cotugno, A. (1996), *Psicodinamica delle relazioni familiari*. Il Mulino, Bologna.

Mantione, M., Presti, F. (2016), "Disturbi sessuali e psicoterapia", in *Disturbi sessuali e psicoterapia, Psicobiettivo, N. 2*, FrancoAngeli, Milano.

Marcus, S.V. (2008), "Phase 1 of integrated EMDR an abortive treatment for migraine headaches", *Journal of EMDR Practice and Research*, Vol. 2(1), pp. 15–25.

Masters, W.H., Johnson, V.E. (1966), *Human Sexual Response*, Little, Brown and Company, Boston.

Masters, W.H., Johnson, V.E. (1970), *Human Sexual Inadequacy*, Little Brown, Boston.

Maxfield, L., Hyer, L.A. (2002), "The relationship between efficacy and methodology in studies investigating EMDR treatment of PTSD", *Journal of Clinical Psychology*, Vol. 58, pp. 23–41.

Mayall, A., Gold, S.R. (1995), "Definitional issues and mediating variables in the sexual revictimization of women sexually abused as children", *Journal of Interpersonal Violence*, Vol. X(1), pp. 26–43.

McGoldrick, T., Begum, M., Brown, K.W. (2008), "EMDR and olfactory reference syndrome a case series", *Journal of EMDR Practice and Research*, Vol. 2(1), pp. 63–68.

Mead, M. (1991), *Maschio e femmina*. Mondadori, Milano.

Melnik, T., Abdo, C.H.N. (2005), "Psychogenic erectile dysfunction: Comparative study of three therapeutic approaches", *Journal of Sex and Marital Therapy*, Vol. 31, pp. 243–255.

Melzack, R., Katz, J. (1992), "The McGill pain questionnaire: Appraisal and current status", in Turk., D., Melzack, R. (eds.), *Handbook of Pain Assessment*, Guildford Press, New York.

Meston, C., Heiman, J. (1998), "Ephedrine-activated psysiological sexual arousal in women", *Archives of General Psychiatry*, Vol. 55, pp. 652–656.

Metz, M.E., Pryor, J.L. (2000), "Premature ejaculation: A psychophysiological approach for assessment and management", *Journal of sex and Marital Therapy*, Vol. 26, pp. 293–320.

Michetti, P., Zampogna, E., Mottola, A. (2009), "Impact of diabetes on sexual dysfunction in men and women: A review", *International Journal of Impotence Research*, Vol. 21(5), pp. 422–428.

Miller, B.C., Monson, B.H., Norton, M.C. (1995), "The effects of forced sexual intercourse on white female adolescents", *Child Abuse and Neglect*, Vol. IX(10), pp. 1289–1301.

Montague, D.K., Jarow, J., Broderick, G.A., Dmochowski, R.R., Heaton, J.P., Lue, T.F., Nehra, A., Sharlip, I.D. (2004), "AUA guideline on the pharmacological management of premature ejaculation", *Journal of Urology*, Vol. 172, pp. 290–294.

Moses, R. (2002), *An Integrative Psychotherapy Approach*, Shapiro, F. (ed.), American Psychological Association, Washington, DC.

Mullen, P.E., Martin, J.L., Anderson, J.C., Romans, S.E., Herbison, G.P. (1996), "The long-term impact of the physical, emotional and sexual abuse of children: A community study", *Child Abuse and Neglect*, Vol. XX(1), pp. 7–21.

Munoz, L. (1991), "Impotencia sexual. Tratamiento conductal con pareja sustituta", *Acta Psiquiatrica v Psicologica de America Latina*, Vol. 37(3), pp. 233–240.

Myers, D.G. (1989), *Social Psychology*, McGraw-Hill, New York.

Nathanson, D.L. (1992), *Shame and Pride: Affect, Sex, and the Birth of the Self*, W.W. Norton & Company, New York.

Nicolosi, A., Glasse, D.B., Moreira, E.D., Villa, M. (2003), "Prevalence of erectile dysfunction and associated factors among men without concomitant diseases: A population study", *International Journal Impotence Research*, Vol. 15(5), pp. 329–336.

Nijenhuis, E.R.S., Spinhoven, P., van Dyck, R., van Der Hart, O., Vanderlinden, J. (1998), "Psychometric characteristics of the somatoform dissociation questionnaire: A replication study", *Psychoterapy and Psychosomatics*, Vol. 67, pp. 17–23.

Nijenhuis, E.R.S., Van Dyck, R., Van der Hart, O., Spinhoven, P. (2003), "Evidence for associations among somatoform dissociation, psychological dissociation, and reported trauma in patients with chronic pelvic pain", *Journal of Psychosomatic Obstetrics and Gynecology*, Vol. 24, pp. 87–98.

Nijenhuis, E. R. S., & Van der Hart, O. (2011). Dissociation in trauma: Elucidation of a psychobiological wound. *Journal of Trauma & Dissociation*, 12(4), 416–445.

Nobre, P.J., Pinto-Gouveia, J. (2003), "Sexual modes questionnaire: Measure to assess the interaction among cognitions, emotions and sexual response", *Journal of Sex Research*, Vol. 7, pp. 48–53.

Nurnberg, H.G., Hensley, P.L., Gelenberg, A.J., Fava, M., Lauriello, J., Paine, S. (2003), "Treatment of antidepressant-associated sexual dysfunction with sildenafil: A randomized controlled trial", *JAMA*, Vol. 289(1), pp. 56–64.

Nusbaum, M.R., Hamilton, C., Lenahan, P. (2003), "Chronic illness and sexual functioning", *American Family Physician*, Vol. 67, pp. 347–354.

Oberlander, L.B. (1995), "Psychological issues in child sexual abuse evaluations: A survey of forensic mental health professional", *Child Abuse and Neglect*, Vol. IX(4), pp. 475–790.

Ogawa, J.R., Sroufe, L.A., Weinfield, N.S., Carlson, E.A., Egeland, B. (1997), "Development and the fragmented self: Longitudinal study of dissociative symptomatology in a nonclinical sample", *Development and Psychopathology*, Vol. 9, pp. 855–879.

O'Hagan, K.P. (1995), "Emotional and psychological abuse: Problem of definition", *Child Abuse and Neglect*, Vol. IX(4), pp. 449–461.

Olson, P.E. (1990), "The sexual abuse of boys: A study of the long-term psychological effects", in Hunter, M. (ed.), *The Sexually Abused Male. Vol. I: Prevalence, Impact and Treatment*, Lexington Books, New York, pp. 137–152.

Ozer, E.J., Best, S.R., Lipsey, T.L., Weiss, D.S. (2003), "Predictors of post-traumatic stress disorder and symptoms in adults: A meta-analysis", *Psychological Bulletin*, Vol. 129, pp. 52–73.

Pagani, S., Di Lorenzo, G., Verardo, A.R., Nicolais, G., Monaco, L., Lauretti, G., Russo, R., Niolu, C., Ammaniti, M., Fernandez, I., Siracusano, A. (2012), "Neurobiology of EMDR – EEG imaging of treatment efficacy", *PLoS One*, Vol. 7, pp. 1–12.

Pagani, S., Di Lorenzo, G., Verardo, A.R., Nicolais, G., Monaco, L., Lauretti, G., Russo, R., Niolu, C., Ammaniti, M., Fernandez, I., Siracusano, A., Fernandez, I. (2011), "Pre-intra-and post-treatment EEG imaging of EMDR-methodology and preliminary results from a single case", *Journal of EMDR Practice & Research*, Vol. 5, pp. 42–56.

Perelman, M.A. (2002), "Sildenafil sex therapy and retarded ejaculation", *Journal for Sex Education and Therapy*, Vol. 26, pp. 13.

Perelman, M.A. (2006), "Psychosocial aspects related to erectile dysfunction", in Mulcahy, J.J. (ed.), *Male Sexual Function: A Guide to Clinical Management. Second Edition*, Humana Press, Inc., Totowa, NJ.

Perry, B.D. (1994), "Neurobiological sequelae of childhood trauma: Post-traumatic stress disorders in children", in Murberg, M. (ed.), *Catecholamine Function in Post Traumatic Stress Disorder: Emerging Concept*, American Psychiatric Press, Washington, pp. 233–255.

Peters, D.K., Range, L.M. (1995), "Childhood sexual abuse and current suicidality in college women and men", *Child Abuse and Neglect*, Vol. 19, pp. 335–341.

Petruccelli, I., Scardaccione, G. (1998), "Violenza sessuale e valutazione del danno psicologico", in *Sessualità e Terzo Millennio. Verso nuovi comportamenti sessuali*, Angeli, Milano, pp. 457–476.

Pourmand, G., Alidaee, M.R., Rasuli, S., Malesi, A., Mehrsai, A. (2004), "Do cigarette smokers with erectile dysfunction benefit from stopping? A prospective study", *BJU International*, Vol. 94(9), pp. 1310–1313.

Protinsky, H., Sparks, J., Flemke, K. (2001), "Using eye movement desensitization and reprocessing to enhance treatment of couples", *Journal of Marital and Family Therapy*, Vol. 27, pp. 157–164.

Putnam, F.W. (2003), "Ten-year research update review: Child sexual abuse", *Journal of the American Academy of Child and Adolescente Psychiatry*, Vol. 42, pp. 269–278.

Pynoos, R.S., Fairbank, J.A, Briggs-King, E., Steinberg, A.M., Layne, C., Stolbach, B.C., Ostrowski, S. (2008), *Trauma Exposure, Adverse Experiences and Diverse Symptom Profiles in a National Sample of Traumatized Children*, International Society for Traumatic Stress Studies, Chicago.

Rajan, A.S., Gopalan, S., Muralidharan, K. (2006), "Sexual dysfunction in women with diabetes: A review", *Journal of Sex & Marital Therapy*, Vol. 32(2), pp. 131–138.

Rhoden, E.L., Morgentaler, A. (2003), "Erectile dysfunction", *Journal of Long-Term Effects of Medical Implants*, Vol. 13(6), pp. 519–528.

Ricci, R.J., Clayton, C.A., Shapiro, F. (2006), "Some effects of EMDR on previously abused child Molesters: Theoretical reviews and preliminary findings", *The Journal of Forensic Psichiatry & Psychology*, Vol. 17(4), pp. 538–562.

Rifelli, G. (2007), "Questione di integrazione", *Sessuologia News*, p. XV-1.

Rimsza, M.E., Berg, R.A., Locke, C. (1988), "Sexual abuse: Somatic and emotional reactions", *Child Abuse and Neglect*, Vol. 12(2), pp. 201–208.

Romanelli, F., Conte, D., Latini, M., Isidori, A. (2000), "Ipogonadismi maschili", in Andreoli, M. (ed.), *Manuale medico di endocrinologia e metabolismo*, Il Pensiero Scientifico Editore, Roma.

Rosen, R.C. (2001), "Measurement of male and female sexual dysfunction", *Current Science*, Vol. 3, pp. 182–187.

Rosen, R.C., Lane, R.M., Menza, M. (1999), "Effects of SSRIs on sexual function: A critical review", *Journal of Clinical Psychopharmacology*, Vol. 19, pp. 67–85.

Roth, S., Newman, R., Pelcovitz, D., van Der Kolk, B., Mandel, F.S. (1997), "Complex PTSD in victims exposed to sexual and physical abuse: Results from the DSM-IV field trial for post-traumatic stress disorder", *Journal of Traumatic Stress*, Vol. 10, pp. 539–556.

Rowland, D.L. (2005), "Psyhophysiology of ejaculatory function and dysfunction", *World Journal of Urology*, Vol. 23, pp. 82–88.

Rowland, D.L., McMahon, C.G., Abdo, C. (2010), "Disorders of orgasm and ejaculation in men", *Journal of Sexual Medicine*, Vol. 7, pp. 1668–1686.

Runtz, M.G. (1997), "The effects of child sexual abuse on adult sexual functioning", *Journal of Interpersonal Violence*, Vol. 12(1), pp. 44–60.

Sachs, B.D. (2003), "The false organic-psychogenic distinction and related problema in the classification of erectile dysfunctions", *International Journal of Impotence Research*, Vol. 15, pp. 72–78.

Schnarch, D. (2000), "Desire problems: A systemic perspective", in Leiblum, S., Rosen, R. (eds.), *Principles and Practice of Sex Therapy*, Guildford Press, New York, pp. 17–56.

Schneider, S.J., Hofmann, A., Rost, C., Shapiro, F. (2008), "EMDR in the treatment of chronic phantom limb pain", *Pain Medicine*, Vol. 9(1), pp. 76–82.

Schore, A.N. (1994), *Affect Regulation and the Origin of the Self: The Neurobiology of Emotional Development*. Lawrence Erlbaum Associates, Hillsdale, NJ.

Schore, A.N. (2001), "Effects of a secure attachment relationship on the development of the right brain", *Attachment & Human Development*, Vol. 3(2), pp. 95–116.

Schore, A.N. (2002), "Dysregulation of the right brain: A fundamental mechanism of traumatic attachment and the psychopathogenesis of posttraumatic stress disorder", *Australian and New Zealand Journal of Psychiatry*, Vol. 36, pp. 9–30.

Schore, A.N. (2003), *Affect Dysregulation and Disorders of the Self*, Norton, New York.

Schuster, T.G., Ohl, D.A. (2002), "Diagnosis and treatment of ejaculatory dysfunction", *Urologic Clinics of North America*, Vol. 29, pp. 939–948.

Sedgwick, E.K., Frank, A. (1995), "Shame in the cybernetic fold: Reading Silvan Tomkins", *Critical Inquiry*, Vol. 21(2), pp. 496–522.

Sehgal, V.N., Srivastava, G. (2003, November–December), "Erectile dysfunction", *SKINmed*, Vol. 2(6), pp. 350–356.

Seidman, S.N., Roose, S.P. (2000), "The relationship between depression and erectile dysfunction", *Current Psychiatry Report*, Vol. 2(3), pp. 201–205.

Sexual Assault Crisis Center of Knoxville (1998), *Child Sexual Abuse*, pp. 1–4, www.cs.edu/barley/sacc/childAbuse.html.

Shapiro, F. (1995), *Eye Movement Desensitization and Reprocessing: Basic Principles, Protocols and Procedures*, Guildford Press, New York – Traduzione in italiano Fernandez, I. (2000), *EMDR. Desensibilizzazione e rielaborazione attraverso i movimenti oculari*, McGraw-Hill, Milano.

Shapiro, F. (1999), "Eye movement desensitization and reprocessing: Clinical and research implications of an integrated psychotherapy treatment", *Journal of Anxiety Disorders*, Vol. 13, pp. 35–67.

Shapiro, F. (2001), *Eye Movement Desensitization and Reprocessing. Basic Principles, Protocols and Procedures. Second Edition*, Guildford Press, New York.

Shapiro, F., Laliotis, D. (2011), "EMDR and the adaptive information processing model: Integrative treatment and case conceptualization", *Clinical Social Work Journal*, Vol. 39, pp. 191–200.

Signorelli, M.S. (2014), "I Disturbi sessuali nel DSM – 5. Aspetti relazionali tra vecchie e nuove diagnosi", *Quaderni di Gestalt*, Vol. 1, p. XXVII.

Simonelli, C. (1997), *Diagnosi e trattamento delle disfunzioni sessuali*, Franco Angeli, Milano.

Simonelli, C. (2006), *L'approccio integrato in sessuologia clinica*, Franco Angeli, Milano.

Simonelli, C., Fabrizi, A., Marciante, N. (1998), "La sessualità femminile tra vecchi clichè e nuovi obblighi", *Rivista di Sessuologia Clinica*, Vol. 2, pp. 51–55.

Simonelli, C., Rossi, R., Forleo, R. (2003), "Le disfunzioni sessuali femminili", in *Encyclopèdie Mèdico Chirurgicale, Ginecologia-Ostetricia. Vol. 166-A-10*, Elsevier, Paris.

Simpson, J.A. (1994), "Attachment and the experience of emotion in adult romantic relationships", *Journal of Social and Personal Relationships*, Vol. 11(1), pp. 43–64.

Simpson, T.L., Westerberg, V.S., Little, L.M., Trujillo, M. (1994), "Screening for childhood physical and sexual abuse among outpatient substance abusers", *Journal of Substance Abuse Treatment*, Vol. XI(4), pp. 347–358.

Soberman, G.B., Greenwald, R., Rule, D.L. (2002), "A controlled study of eye movement desensitization and reprocessing for boys with conduct Problem", *Journal of Aggression, Maltreatment & Trauma*, Vol. 6(1), pp. 217–236.

Solomon, R.M., Rando, T.A. (2007), "Utilization of EMDR in the treatment of grief and mourning", *Journal of EMDR Practice and Research*, Vol. 2(4), pp. 315–325.

Sorrels, K.L., Karpel, M., Roberts, R. (2007), "Sexual dysfunction: An overview", *American Family Physician*, Vol. 75(3), pp. 419–426.

Spinazzola, J., Ford, J.D., Zucker, M., van der Kolk, B.A., Silva, S., Smith, S.F., Blaustein, M. (2005), "Survey evaluates complex trauma exposure, outcome, and intervention among children and adolescents", *Psychiatric Annals*, Vol. 35, pp. 433–439.

Sprang, G. (2001), "The use of eye movement desensitization and reprocessing in the treatment of traumatic stress and complicated mourning: Psychological and behavioral outcomes", *Research on Social Work Practice*, Vol. 11, pp. 300–320.

Steggall, M.J., Gann, S.Y. (2002), "Assessing patient with actual or potential erectile dysfunction", *Professional Nursing*, Vol. 18(3), pp. 155–159.

Sternberg, R.J. (1986a), "A triangular theory of love", *Psychological Review*, Vol. 83, pp. 119–135.

Sternberg, R.J. (1986b), "The nature of love", in Duck, S.W. (ed.), *Handbook of Personal Relationships: Theory, Research and Interventions*. Wiley, Chichester, UK, pp. 173–195.

Sungur, M.Z., Gündüz, A. (2014), "A comparison of DSM-4-TR and DSM-5 definitions for sexual dysfunctions: Critiques and challenger", *Journal of Sexual Medicine*, Vol. 2, pp. 364–373.

Symonds, T., Roblin, D., Hart, K., Althof, S. (2003), "How does premature ejaculation effect a man's life", *Journal of Sex and Marital Therapy*, Vol. 29(5), pp. 361–370.

Terr, L.C. (1991), "Childhood traumas: An outline and overview", *American Journal of Psychiatry*, Vol. 148, pp. 10–20.

Tiefer, L. (2001), "Feminist critique of sex therapy: Fore-grounding the politics of sex", in Kleinplatz, P.J. (ed.), *New Directions in Sex Therapy: Innovations and Alternatives*, Brunner-Routledge, Philadelphia, pp. 29–42.

Tinker, R.H., Wilson, S.A. (2006), "The phantom limb pain protocol", in Shapiro, R. (ed.), *EMDR Solutions: Pathways to Healing*, W.W. Norton & Co., New York, pp. 147–159.

Tripodi, F., Nimbi, F., Fabrizi, A., Rossi, R., Simonelli, C. (2016), "L'approccio integrato in sessuologia", in *Disturbi sessuali e psicoterapia, Psicoobiettivo, N. 2*, FrancoAngeli, Milano.

Uchino, B.N., Cacioppo, J.T., Kiecolt-Glaser, J.K. (1996), "The relationship between social support and physiological processes: A review with emphasis on underlying mechanisms and implications for health", *Psychological Bulletin*, Vol. 119(3), pp. 488–531.

United Nations (2006), *UN Secretary-General's Study on Violence against Children US Department of Health and Human Services*, Agency for Children, Youth and Families.

Urquiza, A.J., Capra, M. (1990), "The impact of sexual abuse: Initial and long-term effects", in Hunter, M. (ed.), *The Sexual Abuse Male. Vol. I*, Lexington Books, New York, pp. 105–135.

U.S. Department of Health and Human Services, Administration for Children and Families, Children's Bureau (2011), *Child Maltreatment 2010*, U.S. Government Printing Office, Washington.

Vaccaro, C.M. (2003), *I comportamenti sessuali degli italiani. Falsi miti e nuove normalità*, Franco Angeli, Milano.

Van der Hart, O., Van Dijk, J., & Steele, K. (1990). "Cognitive-behavioral treatment of traumatic memories." *Journal of Traumatic Stress*, 3(4), 601–620.

van der Hart, O., Nijenhuis, E., Steele, K. (2006), *The Haunted Self: Structural Dissociation of the Personality and the Treatment of Chronic Traumatization*, Norton, New York – Traduzione in italiano (2011), *Fantasmi nel sé. Trauma e trattamento della dissociazione strutturale*, Raffaello Cortina Editore, Milano.

van der Kolk, B. A. (2005). "The effects of trauma on the development of the self." In L. L. C. & A. A. F. N. (Eds.), *The Handbook of Attachment: Theory, Research, and Clinical Applications* (pp. 57–79). New York: Guilford Press.

van Lankved, J., Brewaeys, D., Terkuile, M., Weijenborg, P. (1995), "Difficulties in the differential diagnosis of vaginismus, dyspareunia and mixed sexual pain disorder", *Journal of Psychosomatic Obstetrics & Gynecology*, Vol. 16, pp. 201–209.

Vargo, E.J., Jacobs, A.M. (1988), "The role of sexual dysfunction in the management of chronic illness", *Journal of Psychosomatic Research*, Vol. 32(5), pp. 575–582.

Verardo, A.R. (2016), *Attaccamento traumatico: il ritorno alla sicurezza*, Giovanni Fioriti Editore, Roma, pp. 87–88.

Verardo, A.R., Lauretti, G. (2017), "Protocollo di lavoro con EMDR e sistemi motivazionali nelle relazioni di coppia", *Rivista di Psicoterapia Emdr*, Vol. XI, p. 33.

Waelde, L.C., Koopman, C., Rierdan, J., Spiegel, D. (2001), "Symptoms of acute stress disorder and post-traumatic stress disorder following exposure to disastrous flooding", *Journal of Trauma and Dissociation*, Vol. 2, pp. 37–52.

Waldinger, M.D., Schweitzer, D.H. (2005), "Retarded ejaculation in men: An overview of psychological and neurobiological insights", *World Journal of Urology*, Vol. 23, pp. 76–81.

Waldinger, M.D., Zwinderman, A.H., Putter, H. (2005), "The relationship between erectile dysfunction and depression: A longitudinal study", *International Journal of Impotence Research*, Vol. 17(2), 181–186.

Walker, C.E., Bonner, K.L., Kaufmann, J. (1988), *The Physically and Sexually Abused Child: Evaluation and Treatment*, Pergamon Press, New York.

Webster, L. (1994), "Management of sexual problems in diabetic patients", *British Journal of Hospital Medicine*, Vol. 51, pp. 465–468.

Wiederman, M.W. (1997), "Pretending orgasm durino sexual intercourse in a sample of young adult women", *Journal of Sex & Marital Therapy*, Vol. 23, pp. 75–83.

Wiederman, M.W. (1998), "The state of theory in sex therapy", *The Journal of Sex Research*, Vol. 35(1), pp. 88–99.

Wernik, U. (1993), "The role of traumatic component in the etiology of sexual dysfunctions and its treatment with eye movement desensitization procedure", *Journal of Sex Education and Therapy*, Vol. 19, pp. 212–222.

Winnik, H.Z. (1969), "Second thoughts about 'psychic trauma'", *Israel Journal Psychiatry and Related Disciplines*, Vol. 1, pp. 82–95.

Winson, J. (1993), "The biology and function of rapid eye movement sleep", *Current Opinion in Neurobiology*, Vol. 3, pp. 243–247.

Wodarski, J.S., Jhonson, S.R. (1988), "Child sexual abuse contributing factors, effects and relevant practice issues", *Family Therapy*, Vol. 15(2), pp. 157–173.

Wolfe, D.A., Sas, L., Wekerle, C. (1994), "Factors associated with the development of post-traumatic stress disorder among child victims of sexual abuse", *Child Abuse and Neglect*, Vol. 18(1), pp. 37–50.

World Health Organization (2013), *Mental Health Action Plan 2013–2020*, WHO Press, Geneva.

Zabukovec, J., Huber, A. (1995), "A study of sexual dysfunction in women: The role of psychosocial factors", *Journal of Sex & Marital Therapy*, Vol. 21(1), pp. 33–42.

Zaccagnino, M. (2017), *Nuove prospettive nella cura dei disturbi alimentari. Il ruolo dell'attaccamento nella cura dei disturbi alimentari. Il ruolo dell'attaccamento nel lavoro clinico con EMDR*, Franco Angeli, Milano.

Zaccagnino, M., Cussino, M., Callerame, C., Verardo, A.R., Fernandez, I. (2017), "Effectiveness of EMDR on the attachment internal working models", in *Preliminary Data, to Submit for Publication*.

Zhang, K., He, Z.Y., Xin, Z.C., Jin, J., Guo, Y.L. (2002), "Phisicians'knowledge and attitude to erectile dysfunction", *Zhonghua Nan Ke Xue*, Vol. 8(3), pp. 181–185.

Zilbergeld, B. (1992), *The New Male Sexuality*, Bantam, New York.

Index

Note: Page numbers in *italics* indicate a figure and page numbers in **bold** indicate a table on the corresponding page.